The Vanishing Mind

A SERIES OF BOOKS IN PSYCHOLOGY

Editors:

Richard C. Atkinson
Gardner Lindzey
Richard F. Thompson

The Vanishing Mind

A Practical Guide to Alzheimer's Disease and Other Dementias

LEONARD L. HESTON
University of Washington Medical School
and the
Washington Institute for Mental Illness Research and Training

JUNE A. WHITE
University of Minnesota Medical School

W. H. Freeman and Company
New York

Library of Congress Cataloging-in-Publication Data

Heston, Leonard L.
The vanishing mind: a practical guide to Alzheimer's disease and
other dementias / Leonard L. Heston, June A. White.

p.   cm.
Rev. ed. of: Dementia. 1983.
Includes index.
ISBN 0-7167-2131-7 (hardbound)
ISBN 0-7167-2192-9 (softbound)
1. Alzheimer's disease. 2. Dementia. I. White, June A.
II. Heston, Leonard L. Dementia. III. Title.
[DNLM: 1. Alzheimer's Disease. 2. Dementia. wm 220 h588V]
RC523.H47   1991
362.1'9683—dc20
DNLM/DLC
for Library of Congress   90-15714
                                                              CIP

Printed in the United States of America
1 2 3 4 5 6 7 8 9 0   VB   9 9 8 7 6 5 4 3 2 1

I fear I am not in my perfect mind.
Methinks I should know you, and know this man;
Yet I am doubtful; for I am mainly ignorant
What place this is; and all the skill I have
Remembers not these garments; nor I know not
Where I did lodge last night. Do not laugh at me.

—*King Lear. Act IV, Scene 7*

Contents

Introduction

This book is about a group of diseases that affect the brain. They begin in middle age to late-adult life, and some 30 percent of us will develop one or another of them if we live long enough. The U.S. Congress's Office of Technology Assessment estimates that between 3 and 4 million Americans are currently affected and that the yearly cost to society is 80 billion dollars, which is more than three times the costs associated with heart disease and cancer combined.

These illnesses are widely misunderstood, even by professionals. Because the results are much the same no matter which disease produces them, all are classed together in medicine as *dementias* or *dementing illnesses*. Alzheimer's disease is the best known of the group. What they all produce is a steady, inexorable decline in the function of the brain until death comes, usually eight to ten years after the disease began. Loss of the ability to remember recent events is especially prominent. Those affected cannot learn new material so efficiently as before, and eventually they cannot learn at all. Deficiencies in concentration, judgment, and (often) emotional control become more and more prominent as the disease progresses.

For victims and their loved ones alike, the dementias are devastating. That cannot be glossed over. However, the more families understand about the illnesses facing them, the better they are able to safeguard themselves against their worst effects. So armed, some families even thrive in the face of the dementias. This book is aimed at providing the facts needed to achieve that understanding.

The important questions are intensely practical. How should family members approach an affected person? What medical treatments are available? What is wrong, anyhow? Is it only stubbornness? He or she seems perfectly able to remember some things "when it suits." What about driving? Managing money? Being left alone? Alcohol? Danger because of assaultiveness or carelessness with fire? Should young children and teenagers be exposed to a grandparent affected by dementia? And most important, what can be expected as the disease progresses? Some families know that more than one member has been affected. Is there a genetic component? This book addresses these and many other questions.

Through our professional activities we have become well acquainted with the dementias and with their personal, financial, and societal consequences. For several years our medical research program in the genetics of dementing illnesses has brought us into close contact with families struggling with the dementias. In clinics and hospitals we have been seeing victims of dementing illnesses for diagnostic work-ups and treatment. One of these clinics has been devoted to giving families information about the role of genetic factors in mental illness, including the dementias. In recent years, major activities of this clinic have been determining whether or not persons at risk for Huntington's disease actually possess the pathological gene and counseling them in accordance with the result. Through our experiences we have gained a store of practical information that we believe will be valuable to those who must deal with the dementias. We have aimed our book at the lay reader who will, we think, understand the material readily. Any effort this understanding requires should be rewarded by a good working grasp of the dementias, which will help the reader to plan rationally and ease the burdens of those who suffer from these illnesses and those who love them.

The first edition of this book appeared in 1983 under the title *Dementia*. Since that time much new information has accumulated, so the book has undergone extensive revision. Two areas needed the most attention. First, medical science has continued on its path toward the creation of a revolution as profound as any in the history of our species. In the brain sciences, this revolution is now mainly focused on the molecular mechanisms of gene action and their linkages to consciousness and behavior. The process of discovery is ongoing and far from complete, but our knowledge of the dementing illnesses has benefited through better understanding of their molecular pathology from which has followed important implications for experimental treatments.

Second, profound changes have been occurring in the way society views the dementias and approaches them. Relevant financial, legal, and social institutions have slowly but surely undergone a revolution. We think that we have caught up with these developments and incorporated them into this edition. For example, legislation regarding spousal impoverishment and living wills has helped to preserve the financial solvency of families. Respite care and advocacy organizations such as the Alzheimer's Association have contributed many important new resources.

Our first edition got a most friendly reception, both from those who praised the book without reservation and from those who pointed out deficits. We are grateful to all. Their comments made us especially sensitive to the difficulties that nonprofessionals have with medical science and its jargon. We worked hard to correct that shortcoming because the nonprofessional audience—especially members of affected families—is the one we want most to reach.

Leonard L. Heston
June A. White

CHAPTER 1

Dementia: The Signs and Symptoms

The natural history of a disease—that is, the course it is most likely to follow when no treatment is applied—is as important as anything we can learn about it. Nothing sets the natural history in mind as firmly as a description of a typical case. The following is a composite picture of three persons we knew very well who suffered from dementing illnesses.

Harry: A Victim

Harry seemed in perfect health at age 58, except that for a couple of days he had had the flu. He worked in the municipal water treatment plant of a small city, and there, while responding to a minor emergency, Harry became confused about the order in which the levers controlling the flow of fluids should be pulled. Several thousand gallons of raw sewage were discharged into a river. Harry had been an efficient and diligent worker, so after puzzled questioning, his supervisor overlooked the error. Several weeks later, Harry came home with a baking dish that his wife had asked him to pick up; he had forgotten that he had brought home the identical dish two nights before. Later that month, on two successive nights, he went to pick up his daughter at her job in a restaurant, forgetting that she had changed shifts and was working days. And a week later he quite uncharacteristically became argumentative with a clerk at the phone company; he was trying to pay a bill that he had paid three days before.

By this time his wife had become alarmed about the changes in Harry's behavior. When she discovered that he had been writing little reminder notes to himself on odd scraps of paper, and that these included detailed instructions about how to operate machinery at work if various problems arose, she insisted that he see a doctor. Harry himself realized that his memory had been failing for perhaps as long as a year, and he reluctantly agreed with his wife. The doctor did a physical examination and ordered several laboratory tests and an electroencephalogram (a brain wave test). The examination results were normal, and thinking the problem might be depression, the doctor prescribed an antidepressant drug. If anything, the medicine seemed to make Harry's memory worse. It certainly did not make him feel better. Then the doctor thought that Harry must have hardening of the arteries of the brain, for which there was no effective treatment.

Months passed and Harry's wife was beside herself. Now fully aware of the problem, she could see that it was worsening. Not only had she been unable to get effective help, but Harry himself was becoming resentful and even suspicious of her attempts. He now insisted there was nothing wrong with him at all. She sometimes caught him narrowly watching her every movement, and at other times he accused her of having the police watch him. He would draw all the blinds in the house, and he once ripped the telephone out of the wall; it was "spying." These episodes were tolerable because they were short-lived; besides, there didn't seem to be dangerous intensity to any of Harry's ideas. His wife, who had the summer off from her position as a fourth-grade teacher, began visiting him at his job at least once a day. Soon she was actually doing most of his work; his supervisor, an old friend of the family, looked the other way. Harry seemed grateful that his wife was there.

Approximately eighteen months had passed since Harry had first allowed the sewage to escape, and he was clearly a changed man. He often seemed preoccupied, a vacant smile settled on his face, and what little he said seemed empty of meaning. He had given up his main interests, golf and woodworking. Sometimes he became angry—sudden storms without apparent cause—which was quite unlike him. He would shout angrily at his wife and occasionally throw or kick things, although his actions never seemed intended to hurt anyone. He became careless about personal hygiene, and more and more often he slept in his clothes. Gradually his wife took over, getting him up, toileted, and dressed each morning. Then one day the county supervisor stopped by to tell Harry's wife that Harry just could not work any longer. He would be 62 in a few months and was eligible for early retirement. Of course, he hadn't really worked for a long while anyway, and he had become so inattentive that he was a hazard around machinery.

Harry himself still insisted that nothing at all was wrong, but by now no one tried to explain things to him. He had long since stopped reading; he would sit vacantly in front of the television though unable to describe any program that he had watched. His condition slowly worsened. He was alone at home through the day because his wife's school was in session. Sometimes he would wander out. He greeted everyone he met, old friends and strangers alike, with "Hi, it's so nice." That was the extent of his conversation, although he might repeat ". . . nice, nice, nice. . . ." He had promised not to drive, but one day he took out the family car. Fortunately, he promptly got lost and a police officer brought him home; his wife then took the keys to the automobile and kept them. When he left a coffee pot on the electric stove until it boiled dry and was destroyed, his wife, who by this time was desperate, took him to see another doctor.

Again, Harry was found to be in good health. This time, however, the doctor ordered a "CAT (computed axial tomography) scan." Using this very sophisticated x-ray examination, which we will describe in Chapter 5, the doctor could see that Harry's brain had actually shrunk in size; its diameter was at least 2.5 centimeters (about an inch) less than normal. The doctor said that Harry had "Pick's–Alzheimer disease" and that there was no known cure or treatment.

Harry could no longer be left at home alone, so his daughter began working nights and caring for him during the day until his wife came home after school. Usually he sat all day, but sometimes he wandered aimlessly. He seemed to have no memory at all for events of the day, and he remembered very little of the distant past, which a year or so before he had enjoyed describing. His speech consisted of repeating over and over the same word or phrase, such as, "Hooky then, hooky then, hooky then." His wife tried and tried to find help. She was told the state mental hospitals "did not have a program that would meet his needs." In any case, they could take only committed patients who were dangerous to themselves or others. Harry didn't fit that description.

Because Harry was a veteran, she took him to the nearest Veterans Administration hospital, 150 miles distant. After a stay of nine weeks, during which the CAT scan and all the other tests were repeated with the same results, the doctors said that Harry had a chronic brain syndrome. His wife, who wanted Harry closer to home, found that local nursing homes would charge more than her net monthly salary to care for Harry. Medicare would not pay for nursing home care. However, Social Security and a veteran's pension for which Harry was now eligible would cover about one-third of the charges, bringing the cost barely within the family's financial reach. A visit to the home dismayed her, but she simply could not manage Harry. After a week of indecision, she placed him in the nursing home.

Despite her apprehensions, Harry's wife soon found that the home's staff was competent and professional and that they did their best. Harry was set up in a chair each day, and the staff made sure that he ate enough. Even so, he lost weight and became weaker. When his wife came to see him he would weep, but he didn't talk, and he gave no other sign that he recognized her. After a year he even stopped weeping, and after that, she could no longer bear to visit. He lived on until just after his sixty-fifth birthday when he choked on some food, developed pneumonia as a consequence, and soon died.

Signs and Symptoms

Medical students are warned by their mentors, with a peculiar grim jocularity, to beware of "medical student's disease." As students first learn the signs and symptoms of diseases, they are inclined to discover those signs and symptoms in themselves, their friends, and their relatives—particularly in themselves. The lesson for the students seems simple: "Do not let subjective factors, especially emotions, influence your assessment of signs and symptoms." But in practice, maintaining objectivity can be extremely difficult. This is especially true for those who are trying to be objective about illness in a close relative.

The pitfalls are obvious enough. Dementia begins with forgetfulness, something each of us experiences all too often. When evaluating an instance of forgetfulness, we may, on the one hand, exaggerate its importance and experience a flash of unwarranted worry about ourselves or others, or, on the other hand, minimize it and fail to recognize developing illness. After all, Harry's accident at the water treatment plant and his early lapses of memory are not so different from experiences many of us have had in life. Whereas such occasional lapses are well within the limits of normality, a progressively worsening and irreversible loss of memory signals dementing illness. But it can be very hard to recognize the difference between normal lapses and disease, especially when the disease is just beginning.

The early stages of a dementing illness may be extremely confusing and upsetting for those who are emotionally attached to the victims. Because the early signs are sometimes seen in normal persons and are recognized as evidence of disease only when seen too often or too intensely, we may easily misinterpret them in ourselves or others. Depending on our mood or general outlook, we may exaggerate the importance of failure to remember in ourselves—"Am I getting senile?"—or discount it in others—"he can remember the things he wants to remember." Thus we may find ourselves pulled back and forth, sometimes minimizing, sometimes exaggerating, the significance of what might—or might not—be simple of everyday lapses. This whipsawing is typical, but terribly painful, for families facing dementing illness. Even doctors, who are rigorously trained to counteract subjective, emotion-laden reasoning, sometimes fall victim to it. For the lay person trying to understand a loved one, perfect objectivity is impossible.

Even so, there is much we can do to equip ourselves to distinguish between normal lapses and an early stage of dementing illness. It is especially important to learn to observe carefully and assess four mental functions: memory, judgment, ability to abstract, and emotional responsiveness. In the following sections we take a close look at each one, for deficits in these functions are the symptoms by which we recognize dementia.

Memory

Memory loss such as Harry experienced is so central to dementia, and objective understanding of it is so important, that we will discuss it several times as we proceed. It will therefore be helpful to understand some general features of memory formation. Although much is known about some conditions affecting memory, exactly how it is formed is one of the major unsolved problems of neuroscience and biology. One critical distinction important in dementia is that between short-term (or immediate) memory, and long-term (or distant) memory.

We retain enough information about our immediate environment and its very recent history to enable us to monitor it continuously and adjust our responses accordingly. However, little of this information is stored in long-term memory. Rather, it is quickly forgotten as it obviously must be: There is surely a limit to our storage capacity. For example, we can usually, though sometimes only with effort, recall many details about what we did yesterday afternoon, while what we did a week ago has largely been erased. Long-term memory is first established as short-term memory, and then other brain mechanisms become involved, making it long-lasting. Although the mechanism of this process is unknown, some conditions that govern its regulation, promoting or retarding the formation of long-term memory, are known. Both voluntary and involuntary processes are involved.

We preferentially remember what seems important to us or what we associate with some important emotion or event. For example, if we become ill after breakfast or if, while eating, we learn from the morning paper that we have won a state lottery, we are more likely to remember what we had eaten. We can also establish long-term memory by making special effort. For example, we can memorize nonsense symbols and retain them in memory indefinitely if we make unnatural efforts. We remember important facts for long periods and our memory is helped if the facts are occasionally recalled and used. The vocabulary of a foreign language provides a good example of this process. Emotionally important or stressful events may be retained in long-term memory, whether we want them there or not. Likewise, several factors interfere with the establishment of long-term memory. Emotional arousal appears to inhibit the formation of memories that are not directly related to the cause of the arousal; lovers may be oblivious to everything around them and yet have very intense memories. Alcohol and many other commonly used drugs interfere with memory formation . We will discuss these and other impediments later.

Some dementing illness begins in early middle age and its frequency of occurrence steadily increases thereafter. At any age, the first sign is nearly always loss of recent memory, while long-term memory remains more or less intact. A wedding or a high school football game may be correctly recalled in great detail by a person who cannot retain enough immediate memory to count change after making a purchase. Moreover, the same person may remember an emotionally charged event that occurred a week before, but be unable to converse about the news of the day.

Harry's history illustrates the importance of distinguishing between immediate and long-term memory. He could manage routine operations on his job, but when he had to deal with a minor emergency that required enough recent memory for him to perform effectively while deviating from routine, his disability became evident. Likewise, he managed to pick up his daughter as long as doing so was a familiar routine. When the routine changed, Harry failed to adapt.

Harry's experience at the water treatment plant introduces an important concept, the *threshold*. Our brains and other organs have reserve capacities beyond what is needed to cope with life's ordinary demands. If that reserve capacity is gradually lost to disease, the loss may go unnoticed until a stress (such as the flu) makes added demands, even minor ones, that cannot be met. It is not unusual for a major illness to appear to begin with a flu, as it did in Harry's case, or with some other illness or accident. Then a marginal adaptation may abruptly be lost as a threshold is crossed.

Consider another example. In a normal healthy person, 40 to 45 percent of the volume of blood is taken up by red blood cells that carry oxygen. Given ordinary levels of physical activity, a gradual loss of cells to the point at which they make up a much smaller proportion of the total volume, say 20 to 25 percent, may go unnoticed. But then strenuous activity or an illness, both of which increase the body's requirement for oxygen, may precipitate major signs of illness such as heart failure. A threshold was crossed.

These relationships can be quite confusing for families,

who naturally try to attach a cause to illness. Individuals may wrongly assume or assign guilt for causing illness: "If only I hadn't made him go out in the rain," or "His son was such a worry to him." People seek understandable explanations and too easily accept the one that seems most likely. When seeking to explain illness, they are most often wrong. Keep the threshold perspective when thinking about disease. Challenges to our capacities are a part of normal life. We cannot avoid acknowledging disease by pretending that a challenge caused the problem.

Judgment

Only slightly less noticeable than loss of recent memory as dementing illness progresses is the diminution in the logical and social capacities that we group together and call "judgment." We continuously respond to challenges from our environment. Doing this requires that we obtain information about our environment, integrate it into our consciousness, and make responses or choose not to respond. This is what we mean by judgment.

People with dementia are not able to assimilate information so efficiently as they did before becoming ill, and therefore their responses are less adept. At first, the deficits may be noticeable only in subtle deviations from social deportment; for example, the person may be uncharacteristically inattentive to conversation. She does not grasp the whole context of social situations with the facility she previously exhibited, and hence the quality of her reactions declines. Here too, long-established patterns of behavior that have become in effect automatic tend to be preserved. It is in unfamiliar situations involving new people, new facts, or a new environment that the developing disability is evident.

The relative preservation of old abilities can be deceptive. For example, communication skills tend to be preserved. A verbally fluent person can continue to produce grammatically correct sentences and make use of a large vocabulary despite a moderately advanced dementia. It is only when one looks for the meaning the communication conveys, and compares it with the quality the affected person was previously capable of achieving, that the disability becomes evident.

Ability to Abstract

Closely related to judgment is ability to abstract, and this capacity too declines precipitously. Finding common themes, sorting important details from trivial distractions—these are examples of abstracting abilities that rapidly become impaired. Again, the loss can be difficult to detect in one who has spent a lifetime dealing with abstract ideas. The same words and phrases that served well before illness developed are often repeated and may sound superficially convincing. Only close examination may reveal the underlying vagueness and poverty of thought.

A bedside test that professionals use may help clarify this concept. An examiner instructs: "Name as many four-footed animals as you can." The normal response is to organize the animals into groups: household pets—"dogs, cats, gerbils;" barnyard animals—"cows, horses, pigs;" African wild animals—"lions, zebras, elephants;" and so on. Even a mild degree of dementia interferes with this process and results in fewer responses lacking organization: "dogs and cats, bears, tigers, cows," and so on.

Emotional Responsiveness

Emotionality is yet another major feature of mental life progressively impaired by dementing illness. At first, two conflicting tendencies may be observed in the same person. Decline in emotional responsiveness may lead to an apparently apathetic lack of involvement with events—a flatness of gesture, tone of voice, and facial expression. However, these changes often exist simultaneously with a heightened responsiveness that may be quite alien to personality previously manifest. Increased anxiety in situations previously tolerated, hypersexuality, coarsening of humor, irritability, and sometimes physical striking out may appear. Later, as the disease progresses, apathy and withdrawal come to dominate.

The Course Dementia Follows

Harry exhibited all those major signs of dementing illness. Early in the course of his illness, he sometimes appeared emotionally overreactive (labile in professional jargon). That is, he responded to apparently minor stimuli with tears, increased anxiety, or displays of temper. His temperamental outbursts were ineffective: He didn't hurt anyone because the emotional arousal was short-lived and not really targeted. Harry also became more suspicious, generally *paranoid,* in his outlook. This is a fairly common development in dementia. While it can be quite troublesome, in most cases the erroneous ideas and unfounded suspicions are held only briefly, and actions based on them do not seem to be fueled by dangerous emotional fervor. Later, Harry became totally unresponsive. Over the course of his illness, the changes in his behavior represent unmistakable and irreversible stages in the destruction of his personality.

As Harry's history illustrates, the diseases that cause dementia progress at a fairly steady rate and no periods of improvement intervene. Memory decline remains the salient sign of progressive illness. Although immediate memory remains relatively more severely impaired, long-term memory also eventually becomes affected. A past event may be recalled in response to questions, but the description comes to lack details and finally only unintelligible nonsense phrases are produced. Later, as in Harry's case, members of the immediate family are not recognized. Communication of any kind becomes rarer, and toward the end it effectively ceases. The occasional bursts of emotion give way to a pervasive apathy. The affected person becomes physically less active. More time is spent staring off into vacant space.

Later still, changes in the nervous control of muscles may occur. These changes most often produce rigidity due to increased muscle tone (hypertonicity). Because of this rigidity, help may be needed in daily activities, even bringing food to the mouth. Rigidity may also produce painful cramping, which is often especially troublesome at night. Eventually, the illness advances until the affected person is bedfast.

Two other disturbances of nervous control, seizures and myoclonic jerks, often appear late in the disease. Seizures (epileptic fits) usually take the form of rapid alternating movements of arms, legs, or both. Urine or feces may be involuntarily lost, and generally a brief period of unconsciousness follows. Seizures are alarming to those who are not accustomed to seeing them. However, they are usually quite harmless when they appear as a feature of dementing illness, and they are much less distressing than cramps to the ill person. Myoclonic jerks are abrupt, irregular, and involuntary contractions of muscles that produce jerky movements. These are not painful and are not usually distressing to the affected person. About 50 percent of affected persons develop seizures, myoclonic jerks, or both.

Just before the last stages are reached, there is often a substantial loss of weight. Most victims have to be fed. If loss of bladder and bowel control has not occurred during the previous months, it occurs at this time. Skilled nursing care is generally required to prevent bed sores from becoming a major problem. Death, when it mercifully comes, is not directly due to dementing illness. Pneumonia, kidney infection, and choking on food are three common direct causes. But the predisposition to death is unquestionably brought about by dementia; the real cause is one of the cruelest diseases to assail the human spirit.

CHAPTER 2

Diseases That Produce Primary Dementia

If we were to judge only by his signs and symptoms, Harry's illness could have been due to any one of several diseases that produce dementia. These diseases are the subject of this chapter and the one that follows. It is very difficult to distinguish among these diseases while the affected person is still alive. All the individuals from whose cases we have compiled Table 1, for example, were diagnosed by experienced physicians who knew them well as having Alzheimer's disease or a condition described by some unofficial diagnostic term such as "organic brain syndrome" that has a similar medical meaning. The table presents the distribution of final diagnoses determined by autopsy; each diagnosis was proven by actual pathological changes in brain tissue. In life, any of the people

**Table 1 Actual Causes of Dementia as Determined by
Autopsy of Patients Diagnosed in Life as
Having Alzheimer's Disease**

Causes	Percent of cases
Dementia of the Alzheimer type	45
Multi-infarct dementia	20
Mixed Alzheimer and multi-infarct dementia	10
Pick's disease	5
Infections	3
Other unclassified dementias	17

could have been Harry. Obviously, accurate diagnosis before autopsy is not yet possible.

No matter how difficult, distinguishing among the diseases listed in Table 1 is most important to doctors, patients, and families. Some can be treated or even cured, so they must be recognized without delay. Knowing which is present makes realistic planning possible. Each disease has its own natural history. They differ in average age at onset, in average length of illness, or in other features such as muscular control.

Understanding the dementing illnesses is easier when we first separate them into three groups:

1. Primary undifferentiated dementia. This category includes Alzheimer's disease, Pick's disease, and the "other dementias" category in Table 1. These diseases primarily affect the brain and produce dementia through direct effects on brain tissue. They resemble one another quite closely and generally cannot be distinguished by ordinary diagnostic procedures (this is why they are called undifferentiated). A direct examination of brain tissue, usually obtained by an autopsy, is required for diagnosis. These diseases are the major subject of this book. Harry had one of them.

2. Primary differentiated dementia. The conditions in this category usually, but not always, feature disturbances in muscular control that set them apart from the primary undifferentiated group. Most of them are rare causes of dementia, but we will describe them in order to complete the picture of the dementias that families and doctors encounter. These diseases will also help illustrate important general principles of neurology and genetics.

3. Secondary dementia. The secondary dementias are described in Chapter 3, along with other diseases and conditions that may look like progressive dementia but are not due to impairment of the brain. These conditions can often be successfully treated, so accurate diagnosis is crucial. They include multi-infarct dementia (dementia due to progressive blockage of small brain arteries) and infections.

Primary Undifferentiated Dementias

As we have noted, the primary undifferentiated dementias include dementia of the Alzheimer type (DAT), Pick's disease, and "other dementias."

Dementia of the Alzheimer Type (DAT)

Alzheimer's disease, or dementia of the Alzheimer type, is the most common dementing illness. It affects 20 to 30 percent of those who live into their mid-eighties, males and females alike, and it accounts for about half of the cases of dementia at any age. A German physician, Alois Alzheimer, identified and described the disease named for him in a 1907 article. Dr. Alzheimer described the changes he saw under his microscope in brain tissue removed from a person who had an illness similar to Harry's. Because of their appearance under his microscope, Alzheimer named the changes neurofibrillary tangles and senile plaques. A valid diagnosis of a dementia of the Alzheimer type still requires observation of these same changes in brain tissue. Since we cannot, except in exceptional circumstances, remove a portion of the brain from a living person for examination, we cannot be certain of the diagnosis unless we perform this examination by autopsy. As it happened, Harry's brain did exhibit these changes, and the diagnosis was made.

Let's take a closer look at the brain though a low-power microscope (Figure 1). The brain contains millions of nerve cells with neurofibrillary tangles such as those shown. These tangles are composed of microtubules and microfilaments, which are components of the cytoskeleton (literally, "the skeleton of the cell"). Microtubules and microfilaments normally course symmetrically through nerve cells, providing structural support and transporting nutrients to distant parts of the cell. (Nerve cells may be several feet long.) In Alzheimer's disease, this structural network becomes wildly disorganized. The cytoskeleton appears as a tangled mass: an affected cell cannot be functional and is probably dead.

There are also myriads of another important lesion, the senile plaque. Senile plaques are BB-sized accumulations of debris left over from destroyed neurons that surround a central core of amyloid. Amyloid is a small fragment of a large protein that accumulates in nerve tissue and brain blood vessels in the brains of those who have Alzheimer's disease. It will be seen to play a most important role as the science of this illness unfolds in the following sections.

Senile plaques and neurofibrillary tangles spare some parts of the central nervous system, notably the cerebellum and the spinal cord, but they infest those parts most directly concerned with memory and higher mental functioning. It is also curious (and probably significant if only we understood the biology) that we are the only species affected with neurofibrillary tangles and senile plaques. Some aged animals—dogs and nonhuman primates, for example—develop changes in the brain that are analogous in some respects, but these changes are not quite the same. They also do not have the same anatomic distribution, and only occasional cells are affected.

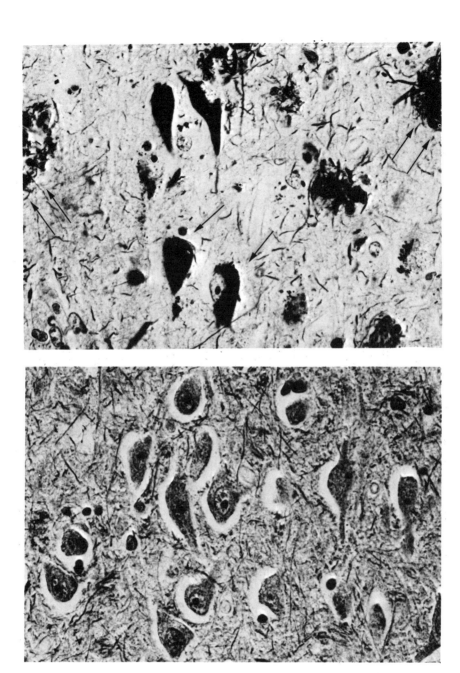

Figure 1 Alzheimer's disease: Microscopic changes in brain tissue.
Above: Brain tissue from a patient with Alzheimer's disease. The single arrows point to neurofibrillary tangles, the double arrows to typical examples of senile plaques. Below: Normal brain tissue containing no such structures. Magnification 550×. *Courtesy of Dr. Angeline R. Mastri.*

The nerve cells, or neurons, that are being destroyed in Alzheimer's disease are the working components of the brain. From them come the commands that set our muscles in motion. They contain our memories, receive the sights and sounds of our surroundings, cause our hormones to be secreted, and produce our emotions. Nerve tissue affected by Alzheimer's disease looks dead. Obviously, a brain containing many neurofibrillary tangles and senile plaques is not functioning well enough to interpret life in all of its richness or to mount a human response to it.

These plaques and tangles are found in human conditions other than Alzheimer's disease, mainly normal aging and Down's syndrome. A few brain cells in most of us will develop such changes if we live to fairly advanced ages—say, into our mid-seventies. Plaques and tangles are widely scattered in ordinary aging, quite unlike the myriads of affected cells seen in Alzheimer's disease. A few such scattered cells do not significantly impair memory or thinking.

In Down's syndrome, or mongolism, plaques and tangles occur in such large numbers that the brain is indistinguishable from that resulting from Alzheimer's disease itself, but the age at onset is much lower, nearly always before age 40. Apparently, a very large proportion of Down's syndrome cases, perhaps approaching 100 percent of those who live to their early forties, develop Alzheimer's changes in their brains and some also develop dementia. It is hard to evaluate intellectual function in Down's syndrome because the individual's skills are severely limited by mental retardation, but even those skills decline. Down's syndrome, which is associated with mental retardation present from birth, may seem oddly out of place when the subject is dementia in otherwise normal adults, but similar changes in the brain suggest a curious link between the two conditions and have provided researchers with valuable clues.

At this point we should clear up some unfortunate confusion in terminology that arose in the years after Alzheimer wrote. The illness that Alzheimer described came to be divided into two diagnostic categories: Alzheimer's disease and senile dementia. In life, the courses of both were similar, and the changes the brain revealed after death were indistinguishable. Nevertheless, the condition was called Alzheimer's disease when the onset of illness was at or before age 65 and senile dementia when the onset was after age 65.

There is an understandable historical basis for this division, and there remain hints that future subtyping of Alzheimer's disease may become necessary. But subdivision requires compelling evidence that two or more diseases actually exist in nature, and today that evidence does not exist. Alzheimer's disease and senile dementia are now regarded as one disease. And over the last few years, both terms have been discarded in formal communication in favor of dementia of the Alzheimer type, (abbreviated DAT) or, senile dementia of the Alzheimer type (abbreviated SDAT). We will use DAT in this book. Pending discovery of evidence to the contrary, we assume the basic disease process is the same, regardless of age at onset.

The age at which DAT begins is, however, a clue to the degree of severity of the illness. In DAT, as in most chronic illnesses, the earlier the onset, the greater the severity. It is very difficult to pinpoint the age at which a dementing illness begins. The onset is insidious. Therefore, by convention, age at onset is operationally defined as the age at which deficits in recent memory first become irreversibly established. In Harry's case, this occurred when his bringing home the second baking dish was closely followed by his failure to remember the change of his daughter's schedule. Such definitions are crude but they are the best available.

Table 2 gives the ages at onset of a series of DAT sufferers who died between 1952 and 1972. Presumably, in a table compiled more recently, today's improved health care would boost the numbers in the "average survival" column, but few data are available. Adding 1.5 years would probably yield a reasonable current estimate. Note that early onset tends to be associated with lesser longevity. Again, this is consistent with medicine's general experience with chronic diseases. The earlier the onset, the more severe the illness, and therefore the

Table 2 Age at Onset Related to Survival in DAT

Age at onset (years)	Percent with onset	Cumulative percent	Average survival (years)	Longest survival (years)
–44	3	3	4.5	6
45–49	2	5	6.1	9.9
50–54	5	10	7.2	12.2
55–59	7	17	8.5	16.1
60–64	14	31	8.4	22.2
65–69	19	50	8.5	18.1
70–74	17	67	8.4	21.3
75–79	18	85	6.1	11.9
80–84	10	95	5.0	13.4
85–	5	100	4.1	8.3

shorter its course. Through the middle range of ages at onset, from 55 to 70, the average time remaining before death was quite consistent—around 8.5 years. Note also that the last column in Table 2, "longest survival," shows survival periods up to 22 years. Though such cases are rare, survival for that long does occur. Onset at more advanced ages is again associated with shorter periods of survival. As age advances, of course, other causes of death (such as cancer or heart disease) become more likely. That effect accounts for the shorter survival periods observed with advanced ages at onset.

As an example of the use of Table 2, suppose that Harry's age at the onset of Alzheimer's disease was 58 years and 6 months. The table reveals that 7 percent of all DAT cases begin between ages 55 and 59, and that Harry was among the 17 percent in whom the disease begins before the sixtieth birthday. The table suggests an average survival of 8.5 years after onset, but to this we must add our "update" correction of 1.5 years making the average estimated survival period 10 years. Harry died 2 years and a few months short of that.

Pick's Disease

In life, Pick's disease appears so much like DAT that attempts to distinguish between the two in living patients have not been successful. An exact diagnosis is possible only by examination of brain tissue, but the differences revealed under the microscope are profound. Figure 2 shows a microscopic slice of brain tissue from an individual who had Pick's disease. Affected nerve cells exhibit Pick's bodies. Like Alzheimer's neurofibrillary tangles, Pick's bodies are masses of neurofilaments and neurotubules in disarray, but their appearance is utterly different from what we saw in Figure 1. Therefore, we must presume that different diseases are present, and that effective treatments, when developed, will likewise be different.

The natural history and course of Pick's disease are not so well known as those of DAT. Average age at onset is estimated as 52.8 years, and death follows after an average of 6.5 years of illness. Survival beyond 8 years is rare in Pick's disease. Table 3 shows how age at onset and severity of illness are related in Pick's disease. And here the table offers an important distinction: After the mid-fifties, new cases of Pick's become infrequent, contributing relatively few new cases of dementia. Both Pick's disease and DAT have occasionally been observed to begin at ages in the early twenties, but that is extremely rare. Females may have a slightly greater risk than males of developing Pick's disease; this is not true for DAT.

A syndrome associated with disease of paired, marble-sized brain centers known as the amygdaloid nuclei, though rare in any illness, may be more frequent in Pick's disease than in other primary dementing illnesses. The main features are overeating, hypersexuality, and a euphoric disposition. "Overeating" understates the behavior. Affected persons stuff anything available into their mouths—food, matches, rubber bands, toilet paper. Choking may become a threat to life. Hypersexuality is usually manifested in self-stimulation; rarely is activity directed at others. The "euphoria" takes the form of a superficial jocularity that usually has no apparent rationale.

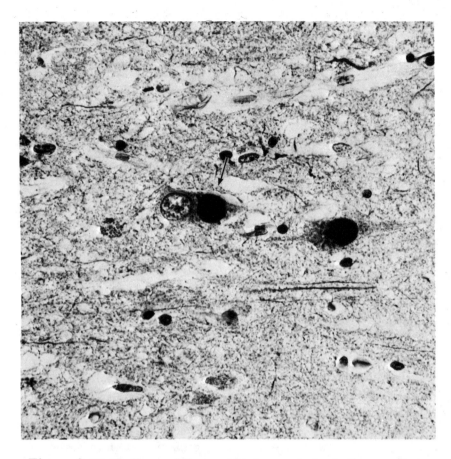

Figure 2 Pick's disease: Microscopic changes in brain tissue.   Brain
tissue from a patient with Pick's disease. The arrow indicates an inclusion
in a nerve cell that is typical of Pick's disease. Note how this brain tissue
differs from that of a victim of DAT (Figure 1). Magnification 550×. *Courtesy
of Dr. Angeline R. Mastri.*

These diagnostic hints can be important. Pick's disease is
much less frequent than DAT at any age, but it remains an
important diagnostic alternative because cases of Pick's disease
are concentrated in age ranges where they are likely to be
confused with those DAT cases that have a relatively youthful

Table 3 Age at Onset Related to Survival in Pick's Disease

Age at onset (years)	Percent with onset	Cumulative percent	Average survival (years)	Longest survival (years)
–39	9	9	4.5	4.5
40–49	12	21	6.9	8.1
50–59	36	57	7.4	8.0
60–69	18	75	7.6	8.8
70–79	9	85	7.2	7.4
80–	15	100	3.4	4.4

onset. As was noted with regard to DAT, youthful onset is associated with relatively more severe diseases, which implies greater risk to relatives and more flagrant biochemical or physiological faults. For these reasons, it is precisely these early-onset cases that are most important to families and medical scientists alike.

Other Dementias of Uncertain Type

A significant proportion of persons who in life exhibited a dementing course indistinguishable from that of DAT or Pick's disease are found upon autopsy to have had neither. They had instead some condition that falls in the category that we will call "other dementias." Table 4 gives the estimated relative frequencies of DAT, Pick's disease, and other dementias according to age at onset.

The "other dementias" are of particular importance, because many of them begin in the middle decades of life and hence are easily confused with Pick's disease and early-onset DAT. Given a case of primary dementia and a reasonably accurate estimate of age at onset, one can obtain from Table 4 an estimate of the probability that the patient is suffering from

**Table 4 Percentages of Primary Dementias with Onset in
the Indicated Age Intervals**

Age at onset (years)	Probability		
	DAT	Pick's	Other dementias
–59	59	21	20
60–69	79	10	11
70–79	90	3	7
80–	97	—	3

each of the of the three listed conditions. For example, a case with onset at age 59 or earlier has a probability of 0.59 (59 percent) of being DAT, 0.21 of being Pick's disease, and 0.20 of being one of the "other dementias."

These proportions are important. Because diagnosis through direct examination of brain tissue is so difficult to obtain, much of the research in the dementias has been based on the assumption that DAT constitutes such a high proportion of all dementias that other causes can safely be neglected. Table 4 makes it clear that this is just not so. Moreover, the stakes are high. All medical experience says that when tissue changes are as distinctive from one another as illustrated in Figures 1 and 2 for DAT and Pick's disease, different causes are at work and different treatments will be effective. Lumping all dementias together is doomed to lead to false conclusions. When evaluating research results, the reader must always ask "How was the diagnosis established?"

The "other dementias" group can be divided into two subgroups. One subgroup, which seems to account for about 60 percent of those dementias, consists of diseases and conditions that are simply unclassified. Examination of some brains representing this group may disclose pathological changes, but they conform to no recognized pattern. Other brains appear entirely normal despite the dementia present in life. The remaining 40 percent of these dementias are known brain diseases distinguished from the primary undifferentiated dementias by features usually—but not always—observable in life. These features are mainly abnormal movements. The diseases are important to medicine and to those directly concerned with dementing illness for two reasons. Sometimes their distinguishing features are absent or not prominent,which may lead to mistaken diagnoses of DAT or Pick's disease. Also, this group of diseases provides useful examples of brain function and genetic principles.

Normal-Pressure Hydrocephalus (NPH)

This important disorder, which is also known as low-pressure hydrocephalus (LPH), or "water on the brain", may account for as many as 5 percent of mid-life dementias. It occupies an uncertain position with respect to the diseases we have so far considered, but we regard it as more closely related to the primary undifferentiated dementias than to any other diagnostic group.

In 1968, psychiatrists and neurologists were cheered by news that the cause of a form of dementia had been discovered and, better yet, that this dementia was treatable by a surgical operation. Doctors eagerly searched for patients who matched the published descriptions. Some were found and operated on to their great benefit. Hydrocephalus clearly does cause some dementias, and surgical treatment is indeed effective. The early optimism, however, has been greatly tempered by unhappy results in a significant proportion of cases.

Normal-pressure hydrocephalus (NPH) involves impaired circulation of spinal fluid. Cerebrospinal fluid (often abbreviated CSF) is a clear, colorless fluid related to lymph. It is secreted into compartments within the brain called ventricles; these are filled with CSF. There are four ventricles—two small and midline in the brain, two large and on either side of the midline. The latter two are called lateral ventricles. CSF is secreted within the lateral ventricles, moves rearward through the midline ventricles, and then passes through three small apertures to the outer surface of the brain. It bathes the surface of the brain and the spinal cord and is finally reabsorbed by special structures on the surface of the brain. These return it to the circulating blood through veins that drain into the jugular vein.

Several diseases are produced by disturbance of the production, circulation, or reabsorption of CSF. Hydrocephalus can be produced by obstruction of flow between the places where CSF is produced in the lateral ventricles and where it is absorbed on the surface of the brain. When this occurs, pressure is increased, at least initially, between the lateral ventricles and the obstruction. This pressure destroys brain tissue and, in infants, may even deform the skull. In NPH there is no mechanical obstruction to the flow of CSF and hence no increase in fluid pressure. The pressure is normal (or, compared to the pressures present in obstruction, even low); hence the names given the condition.

There are at least two types of NPH. One type occurs following injury or infection, sometimes years later. In such cases, the hydrocephalus may be due in part to impaired absorption of CSF resulting from destruction of tissue by the original injury. This often occurs after a hemorrhage of blood into the CSF, but the mechanism is by no means completely understood. At any rate, the onset of dementia is not unlike Harry's, but the progression is usually more rapid, and there is a history of previous injury to the brain. In addition, and most important, NPH tends strongly to produce disturbance in standing and walking ("station" and "gait" to the neurologist), urinary incontinence, or both. These problems arise early in the course of the illness. Gait disturbance and incontinence may appear in DAT, Pick' disease, and other primary dementias, but they generally do so quite late in the course of those illnesses.

Dementia, gait disturbance, and incontinence also mark a second type of NPH. This type produces much the same effects, but there is no preceding injury to the brain. There is a further important difference between the two types of NPH. The type that follows injury can benefit greatly from surgery. A small plastic tube is inserted, and through it CSF flows directly from the ventricles to the jugular vein, bypassing the structures that absorb CSF. NPH that develops in the absence of injury does not so often benefit from surgery, and because the surgery itself is risky, the decision to operate must be carefully considered by the operating surgeons, together with patients and their relatives.

NPH can be diagnosed satisfactorily in life, and, because it is one of the few treatable causes of dementia, doctors are very sensitive to the possibility that it is present. The odds therefore favor correct diagnosis and treatment. The history of injury and the appearance of a disturbance in gait early in the course of illness are two important keys to correct diagnosis.

Usually Differentiated Dementias

These conditions produce a dementia, but it is usually accompanied by other features of illness that set it off and allow a diagnosis to be made in life. Although these diseases are individually rare, they are important for two major reasons. Sometimes diagnoses is difficult because the usual distinguishing features do not develop. Then these diseases can easily be confused with an undifferentiated dementia. Second, these diseases illustrate principles that are applicable to all dementias.

Huntington's Disease

Huntington's disease is nearly always distinguished from other dementias by peculiar involuntary writhing movements that any physician can recognize in their typical form. Except that the diagnosis is usually easily made, Huntington's disease has much in common with the undifferentiated dementias, and most of what we shall say about them is also applicable to Huntington's disease.

Viral Illnesses

Creutzfeldt–Jakob disease is an infectious disease that is due
to a virus. It can generally be distinguished from other dementias by its relatively rapid course—months rather than years
from onset to death—but this is not always the case. Some
times the course is prolonged, and, for that matter, some
nonviral undifferentiated dementias progress rapidly. Again,
conclusive diagnosis requires an autopsy.

Two other viral illnesses share important features with
Creutzfeldt–Jakob disease: kuru, which was once endemic
among native groups in New Guinea; and Gerstmann–
Sträussler syndrome, a rare illness without known geographic
boundaries. Although transmission by viral-like agents has
been demonstrated for all three of these illnesses, several cases
occur in some families while other family members, apparently
equally exposed to any infection within the family, escape
illness. This pattern suggests that genetic factors may play a
part in their occurrence. This would not be unusual; genetic
predisposition to viral illness seems to be fairly common. However, the biological principles are complex. We will return to the
subject when we discuss genetic illness.

Other Conditions

There remain miscellaneous dementias that are individually
rare. Some have been described in only one family. One relatively frequent illness of this sort, progressive supranuclear
palsy, might be confused with an undifferentiated dementia.
Paralysis of certain eye movements (upward gaze) is a constant
feature that distinguishes it from other dementias. This illness
is probably related to Parkinson's disease, which is yet another
condition that may include a progressive dementia among its
manifestations. Characteristic tremor, rigidity, and other
neuromuscular features usually (but not always) separate
Parkinson's disease from dementing brain diseases.

Wilson's disease is another malady that may produce a
progressive dementia. Nearly all cases of this rare illness begin

with signs of liver disease. If the brain is involved, impairments of movement are typically the first signs. However, if mental processes deteriorate early in the course, confusion with primary dementia can occur. A competent medical examination should yield a correct diagnosis in even the most unusual case.

This completes the list of brain diseases associated with progressive dementia that might possibly be confused with a primary undifferentiated dementia such as DAT or Pick's disease. Over the last few years, researchers have improved diagnostic accuracy by adopting specific criteria for the diagnosis of DAT, thereby separating this most frequent disease of the group from all the others. This process has reduced the error of overinclusion (false positive diagnoses) to 10 to 15 percent, a level that is hardly ideal but is satisfactory for some research purposes. However, problems remain. The diagnostic criteria are designed for application by major medical centers. Physicians with limited resources may be unable to apply them rigorously. Also, an unknown (but doubtless large) proportion of true cases are excluded from research groups by rigid diagnostic criteria: These are called false negatives. False negatives may well be seriously biasing research groups in unknown directions.

Our discussion of diagnostic considerations does not end here. In the next chapter, we take up diseases and conditions that may produce a dementia or apparent dementia not directly due to brain disease. Because the brain is not the seat of disease, the dementia is called secondary. Equally important, one of these diseases may act in conjunction with brain disease that was already present but producing no noticeable effects or minimal ones: Neither disease alone significantly impairs mental efficiency, but together they may sum to cross a threshold. Exploring this possibility is another key aspect of Chapter 3.

Diseases and Conditions Associated with Secondary Dementia

In Chapter 2, we examined the diseases that produce primary dementia, that is, dementia due to impairment of the brain. Signs of dementia may also be associated with diseases that do not usually attack the brain directly. Disease in most organs of the body can produce significant effects on brain function. Heart and lung diseases are especially important in this respect. Many drugs and toxic substances can also seriously interfere with brain function. These conditions are important because they can mimic many effects of the primary dementias. Moreover, disease of other organs and the effects of drugs may add to the impairment produced by primary brain disease, turning a mild impairment into an incapacitating one. (Remember Harry's flu.) Doctors and concerned nonprofessionals alike are better able to help patients with signs of dementia when they understand these possibilities. Finally, some diseases of the brain itself that do not actually produce dementia may closely mimic dementia. Depression is one of these, and we will begin our discussion with it.

Depression

Depression, a psychiatric disorder, is one of the most common major illnesses of adult life. It can mimic dementing illness so closely that distinguishing between the two disorders is extremely difficult. In fact, some persons who are only depressed die in institutions or nursing homes after years of illness wrongly regarded as dementia. This is rare, however, and because depression is very common, such cases represent a vanishingly small proportion of the total number of depressed persons. Moreover, unrecognized cases tend not to be textbook examples but rather are those "left over" after nearly all depressions have been recognized by treating physicians. In a sense, the sheer numbers of the depressed make errors inevitable. Approximately 30 percent of the population over age 65 will experience a major depression sometime during the next three years. In such a large population, some depressed people will exhibit atypical symptoms, some of which will resemble very closely those of dementia. Mistaking even a few depressions for dementia represents a very tiny percentage error; it is understandable, given human limitations. But we must aim for no error at all, because today, complete recovery from depression is not only possible; it is the rule.

Other considerations complicate the diagnostic dilemma. Dementing illness usually features a depression sometime during its course. This often appears in the early stages, and it can be quite severe. Furthermore, some of the prescription and over-the-counter drugs taken by depressed persons may cause impairments of intellectual functioning that can easily be con-

fused with dementia. In difficult cases, a specialist must be called on, and sometimes even experts cannot arrive at a conclusive diagnosis. Then doctors may advise that treatment for depression be started in the hope that it may be beneficial. This advice is not reckless, but rather reasonable, because depression can be treated successfully whereas most dementias cannot. Not only physicians, but all concerned must give the benefit of diagnostic doubt to the *treatable* condition.

Both depression and dementia are illnesses wherein the participation of families is crucial to both diagnosis and treatment. The more families know, the better they will be able to help the diagnostic process along and to gauge its effectiveness. Therefore, we will examine depression in some depth.

Depression is a disorder of mood. By mood we mean the prevailing "feeling tone" a person experiences over a lengthy period of time—days rather than hours. Climate provides an apt analogy. We may correctly describe a climate as rainy and yet not be surprised at occasional sunshine. Similarly, a depressed mood is perfectly congruent with flashes of normality or even happiness. What counts is the average over a longer time. Variation in mood is normal of course. When good fortune befalls us, our mood tends to be high, just as bad luck occasions a gloomy outlook. If prolonged misfortune or an extremely sad event occurs—the death of a loved one, for example—the low mood is likely to be deeper and longer lasting.

These normal variations are part of our common experience, and we easily understand when we observe them in others: "If that event (or those events) had happened to me, I would be just as low." We generally are not aware of making such an explicit test, but that appears to be the process we follow in assessing feeling states in others. It is not so easy, however, to put ourselves in the place of depressed persons and to assume their perspective. Depressions—and especially the most serious ones—usually occur without any antecedent event. They are described as endogenous, which means that they arise in the absence of sufficient external cause.

When depression is used as a medical diagnosis, the mood change it reflects either (1) is greater than could reasonably be explained as a normal reaction to an external event or (2) has lasted longer than usual after such an event. For example, the death of a spouse commonly produces a deeply depressed mood and is certainly sufficient explanation for such a change. However, the bereaved person's mood should start to lighten after a few weeks, and although intense pangs of depression may be felt for years with decreasing frequency (though not decreasing intensity), the individual's mood should be effectively normal after a few months. Depressive illness should be suspected if these limits are exceeded.

Mood tends to color all of our perceptions. In depression, gloom colors all our judgments and values. Our past memories, our future expectations, our families, our associations—everything we are seems blackened to a degree which depends on the depth of the depression. Every real fault is exaggerated, and many more are imagined. Negativism, guilt, and remorse preoccupy our thinking. One doctor, after recovering from a depression, flatly stated that he could not imagine a more painful disease except perhaps rabies, a disease notorious among professionals for the pain it inflicts.

Mood is a subjective state. We can describe our own mood (though sometimes with difficulty), but we must be told what mood others are experiencing. Their report is the only direct evidence available to us. However, several indirect indicators of mood exist. The affected person seems preoccupied with negative aspects of his or her life. The gloom we have noted usually dominates conversation. The facial expression is sad most of the time. Don't be deceived by a few smiles. We smile through tears almost as much as we smile for joy, because smiling is such a ubiquitous, nonspecific human response. Depressed people often do not have the appetite to eat enough, and weight loss can be quite substantial: The loss of 10 to 20 percent of body weight over a few weeks is not unusual. There is often difficulty sleeping, especially sleeping through the night. A depressed person may go to bed at ordinary times and fall asleep without undue difficulty but may then awaken after an hour or two and be unable to go back to sleep. Those early morning hours are the worst. In general, depression is at its worst on first awakening in the morning and then gets better as the day wears on (the opposite is true in dementia). By early evening, the mood may be nearly normal, even in severely ill persons.

It should be clear by now that a typical depression could hardly be confused with dementia. The problem that arises in diagnosis is due to a small minority of depressions that feature severe retardation. Retarded depression is so named because responses such as movements, thinking, and speech are slowed, often dramatically so. Sometimes there is hardly any speech. Words are separated by such long pauses any continuity may be lost for the listener. This, coupled with a vacant, unchanging facial expression and a generalized poverty of responses, can make the illness look like dementia. Sometimes there is an even more deceptive feature: An actual intellectual deficit may affect memory, abstracting ability, and judgment. Successful treatment of depression reverses these deficits, but without treatment, they much resemble early signs of dementia.

Because of these similarities, depressions may slip by a cursory medical examination, but not a competent one. And even if a depression goes unrecognized, the passage of time usually brings enough improvement to eliminate dementia from consideration. Over a couple of months, many persons afflicted with depression improve and even recover, whereas those with dementia do not improve and may worsen. But simply waiting may mean months of suffering from a treatable illness. And some depressives do not recover spontaneously but rather go on for years without much change.

Although competent physicians can separate depressions from dementias, they rely on descriptions of the course of the illness and the history. In the case of dementia or depression, relatives have to supply much of this history. In Table 5 we have listed the features that we believe are most useful in making the necessary distinctions. The list is by no means exhaustive, but it does include the signs most likely to be noticed by family members.

Table 5 Signs and Symptoms That Help Distinguish Depression from Dementia

Depression	Dementia
Uneven progression over weeks	Even progresion over months or years
Complains of memory loss	Attempts to hide memory loss
Often worse in morning, better as day goes on	Worse later in day or when fatigued
Aware of and exaggerates disability	Unaware of or minimizes disability
May abuse alcohol or other drugs	Rarely abuses drugs

A major distinction between depression and dementia is in the "daily rhythm" of the disorder. In depression, the morning is usually the worst time. Spirits and energy tend to improve as the day wears on. This is by no means always pronounced, and it may not be observable at all, but the opposite pattern is extremely rare. By contrast, dementia worsens notably with increasing fatigue and is therefore most apparent toward the end of the day. Another feature worth noting is the tendency of depressed persons, especially elderly depressed persons, to attempt to medicate themselves with alcohol and drugs. In dementia, drug use seems to decline. Even alcoholics undergoing a dementing process tend to reduce their intake. This tendency is pronounced enough so that increased use of alcohol or drugs points to depression as the first diagnosis to consider.

We have examined depression closely as a disease of the brain that can mimic dementia. Several disorders that are not primarily diseases of the brain, and certain other conditions, can also be confused with dementia or can aggravate the effects of any actual dementing illness. The rest of this chapter is devoted to these diseases and conditions.

AIDS

Over the past five years, a new disease, AIDS (acquired immune deficiency syndrome), has been added to the roster of those producing brain disease that can closely mimic progressive dementia. In the United States, AIDS began as a disease limited mainly to homosexual males, but it soon spread to users of intravenous drugs and to recipients of contaminated blood. The incidence of the disease is increasing in the population at large, and there is no way to know how far it will spread. In 1989 it was the eleventh most frequent cause of death in the United States, and it will certainly be among the top ten by the time you read this description. Although it has tended to be a disease of younger age groups, this will not remain true because those at risk are growing older. During the first six months of 1990 , 10 percent of new cases were in people age fifty or older.

The brain disease produced by AIDS may be mild or severe, and the primary results of brain tissue involvement can be hard to separate from the secondary results of infections and tumors that AIDS produces in other organs, but every AIDS case entails brain disease. The earliest manifestations are malaise, apathy, and a slowing of mental processes. Intermittent loss of recent memory, difficulty in concentrating, and disordered progression of thought follow. Mood disorder or paranoia may occur, but intellectual defects predominate. These signs of brain disease may precede the development of disease in other organs. Because these symptoms resemble those of progressive dementia, a test for the AIDS antibody may soon be required when dementia is being considered as a diagnosis.

Blood Vessel Disease

If AIDS is the disease that has most recently been found to cause brain disease mimicking dementia, blood vessel disease has perhaps been associated with dementia the longest, though not always accurately. Such vascular disease—often called arteriosclerosis or hardening of the arteries—affects the arteries that bring blood to the brain. Until the last two decades, this disease was regarded as the cause of nearly all dementia. We now know that this is not true and estimates of the frequency of dementia due to vascular disease are steadily decreasing. Even so, perhaps 10 to 15 percent of dementias that take a course resembling Harry's are due to blood vessel disease. Moreover, vascular disease can often be successfully treated, so correct diagnosis is extremely important.

The most common form of vascular disease results in an interruption of the blood supply to the brain. The effects rarely resemble those of dementia of the Alzheimer type (DAT) and the other dementias. The brain, which uses a large proportion of the oxygen and sugar available to the body, is extremely sensitive to any shortage or absence of these vital nutrients. Blood carries nutrients to the brain. Brain cells in a middle-aged person can survive only a minute or two without oxygen, and they can live only slightly longer without glucose, the form of sugar most efficiently used by the brain. A stroke is an interruption in the blood supply that continues long enough to damage the brain.

Severity varies. Much depends on the size of the affected blood vessel. Blockage of a large artery carrying blood to a correspondingly large area of the brain can produce massive damage. Such a severe stroke could hardly be confused with a primary dementia. In addition to intellectual functions, voluntary movements and other functions such as speech are affected. Because an artery generally fails over a short period of time, the onset of disability is abrupt, not gradual as in primary dementias. Also, because arteries are generally paired, each member of the pair supplying one side of the body, damage is usually confined to one side of the body. Obviously, paralysis of part of one side of the body and impairment of speech or consciousness indicate a stroke, not dementia.

Sometimes however, the damage is confined to very small arteries. In this case, no one stroke may have any observable effect on movement or intellectual functioning. But when several occur over time, and they are scattered among several small arteries, dementia may develop gradually and may become the major observable sign of an impaired brain. This condition is called multi-infarct dementia. Most often the disability progresses in a series of small steps, each corresponding to the blockage of yet another artery, and then recovery seems to occur. This is an important distinction. Brain tissue can recover, at least partially, from the damage produced by strokes, but it does not recover from the damage produced by the primary dementias. Jerky progression, featuring abrupt worsening followed by gradual partial recovery, is characteristic of vascular disease. However, this idealized course may be hard to recognize in some cases, and in these cases, the course of vascular disease may be hard to distinguish from that of dementing illness.

Certain treatable diseases may predispose people to strokes and multi-infarct dementia: These include high blood pressure, diabetes, and a few rare inflammations of arteries. Measurements of blood pressure and blood sugar should be part of any routine medical checkup and are essential in any investigation of dementia. Inflammation of arteries usually produces other effects (kidney damage, for example), but some forms can be confined to the brain. The erythrocyte sedimentation rate, or "sed rate," which is a simple, routine laboratory measurement, is generally elevated when one of the vascular diseases is present.

About 10 percent of persons with DAT also have significant vascular disease of the brain that warrants a diagnosis of "mixed Alzheimer's and multi-infarct dementia." Some of these cases are due to the actual presence of the two diseases. Somewhat more frequent, we believe, is a complication of a single disease, DAT. Amyloid is found both in senile plaques and in brain blood vessels that it narrows or blocks.

Other Secondary Dementias

Many medical problems besides depression, AIDS, and vascular disease may mimic primary dementia. Such problems may cloud the diagnostic picture and must be rigorously excluded before final diagnostic conclusions are reached. But just as important, diseases and conditions unrelated to an existing brain disease may make an otherwise inconsequential or mild impairment worse. In such cases, the appearance of severe dementia may lead to a premature diagnosis of primary dementia. The major disability is actually due, however, to the combination of mild dementia and some other, possibly correctable problem.

Far too many illnesses may have secondary effects on mental functioning for us to discuss each one separately. Happily, certain general principles can be expressed briefly, which make explanations manageable and simplify understanding.

The condition and functioning of the brain is affected by the condition of the rest of the body. For example, infections anywhere in the body may produce toxins (poisons) that have effects on other parts of the body, including the brain. We have all had viral infections. Our joints may ache, we may feel undue fatigue, and our tempers may be short because of "colds" or "flu," which seem to affect the whole body. Here the cold, a disease of the respiratory system, is affecting other organs, including the brain. Ordinarily such infections present no special problem though we may complain bitterly and even joke that we would rather be dead. However, miserable as we might be, neither our friends, nor we ourselves, could ever confuse such an illness with dementia. Yet that confusion *can* occur when an otherwise innocuous additional stress challenges a brain already affected at subthreshold levels with a progressive disease.

The threshold concept, to which we have now returned, is important enough to warrant restatement. In normal aging, there is a steady decrease in the functional capacity of all organs, including the brain. Apart from the sort of "creakiness" we associate with aging, this decline may not be apparent in day-to-day observation. To be sure, older people may be forgetful; this common condition, called benign senescent forgetfulness, is considered normal. But it is a result of a decrease in the reserve capacity of the brain. We begin life with a most valuable excess capacity in our organ systems. In general, we would hardly miss one kidney, or one gonad, or a length of intestine, or even a sizable hunk of heart muscle. But when presented with extraordinary demands, a system that has little remaining reserve capacity might not be capable of a fully effective response. This can happen to the brain when the "extraordinary demand" is no more than a mild case of the flu.

Infections affect the brain in two basic ways. Acute infections (such as pneumonia, which features fever and abrupt, dramatic onset) sometimes produce delirium. Those affected are obviously severely ill and seem at least intermittently to be out of their heads, unsure where they are or why they are there. Persons of any age can become delirious, but older persons are especially likely to develop chronic smoldering infections that begin and progress insidiously, not obviously doing dramatic damage. Infections of the urinary system (kidneys, bladder, and prostate gland), the respiratory system (especially chronic bronchitis), and chronic abscesses are especially troublesome. Superimpose such an infection on a brain, with little reserve capacity, and, rather than delirium, the result may be inattentiveness, difficulty in concentrating, and apathy that looks frighteningly like dementia. Searching for chronic infection and eliminating any that is found can be difficult, but it must be done because success can produce dramatic improvement in brain function.

Hormone imbalances are another fairly common contributor to disturbed brain function. The thyroid gland sets the operating level of all body processes. Without sufficient thyroid hormones, all tissues (including the brain) function sluggishly. The result is a generalized slowing down that may be difficult to distinguish from dementia—the more so because the onset of the disability that arises from hormone imbalance is ordinarily insidious, and the progression lacks clearly distinguishing features.

The thyroid gland is controlled by the pituitary gland. Erroneous instruction from the pituitary may cause decreased secretion of thyroid hormones and can produce effects similar to those of thyroid insufficiency. The pituitary controls many other hormones as well as the thyroid. Manifestations of pituitary insufficiency are therefore more complex, though the overall effects can again be quite similar to those of dementia.

Drugs

Drugs present extremely difficult and complex problems to those dealing with brain disease. The use of drugs is widespread, and the age groups subject to dementing illnesses are by no means exempt. Drugs influence brain function, and nearly always adversely. They can even mimic the effects of a dementing illness. Their usual action, however, is to add to the impairment of a marginal brain, tipping the balance to overt dysfunction. This is a common and most important problem of middle and late adult life.

The importance of keeping drugs in mind when trying to understand and cope with dementia cannot be overstated. When signs of dementia appear, those concerned should think first of drugs. A knowledgeable doctor always inquires carefully into drug use and may ask relatives to search the affected person's living quarters and bring in all the drugs they find. No one should be surprised or offended by such requests, or by the physician's ordering the testing of urine, blood, or both for traces of drugs. These tests have become extremely efficient. One sample of blood and urine is sufficient to screen for even very small amounts of some dozens of drugs likely to produce problems.

Learning about drugs is easier when we take them up in pharmacologic groups. Sedatives, narcotics, stimulants, and hallucinogenic agents are all subject to overuse and voluntary abuse. Other drugs are prescribed, usually for some specific therapeutic purpose, and are generally not abused. But these drugs, too, may cause severe problems. Let's look at each of these five categories in turn.

Sedatives

By far the most important group of drugs for older Americans are the sedatives: alcohol, antianxiety agents such as Valium and Librium, and drugs that promote sleep, such as barbiturates. Two distinct effects phases of drug use may cause serious problems—taking the drugs and undergoing withdrawal from them.

Sedative drugs produce relaxation and intoxication, which most people find enjoyable in their mildest stages. Many people use alcohol daily, often in the form of an evening "cocktail hour." Moderate and controlled use of alcohol is a part of life for millions of us, and most often it is a pleasurable and harmless part. Yet there is a darker side. Too much of any sedative drug produces adverse effects: Severe intoxication (drunkenness) is all too familiar in our society. Addiction and chronic mild intoxication are also common though not so easily recognized.

The amount of a sedative drug that one can take without becoming intoxicated diminishes slowly with age because of a combination of age-related impairments. The liver, which disposes of most drugs, cannot do so as efficiently; because increased age means less body water, drugs (alcohol for one) that are distributed uniformly in body water become more concentrated; because there are fewer brain cells, the effects of drugs on those remaining may be greater; and so on. Most often these factors have little practical effect. People adjust their intake slowly as they age, and the reserve capacity of most organs is great enough to prevent overt problems.

It is a different matter when the brain becomes compromised; then any added challenge may prove calamitous. All sedative drugs interfere with the formation of memory. Thus an alcoholic drink or two may act on an impaired brain to produce signs of dementia. If light drinking occurs throughout much of the day, as is often the case, memory may be seriously impaired for long periods. Moreover, the use of several sedative drugs is not uncommon—for example, a dose or two of Valium during the day and a few drinks at night. The effects add up.

Severe problems may also arise when people who have been taking sedative drugs stop taking them. Withdrawal may induce increasing agitation, perhaps delirium, and even seizures. It can be life-threatening, and it certainly requires medical supervision. Mental problems caused by withdrawal from sedative drugs are nearly always easily recognized. There are, however, two drugs that produce unusually severe withdrawal symptoms in some persons, even when the dosage has been moderate. These are Doriden (glutethimide) and Placidyl (ethchlorvynol). Withdrawal from either can produce puzzling and long-lasting signs of impaired brain function. Although these signs usually resemble those of delirium more than of dementia, the whole picture is a confused one. Distinctions are hard to make, especially when withdrawal is superimposed on a brain that is already compromised.

Narcotics

Popular lore might lead one to think that narcotic drugs such as morphine, codeine, dilaudid, and Percodan, and synthetic drugs such as Darvon would gravely complicate the signs of dementing illness, if not mimic them precisely. But this is not so. These drugs are, of course, commonly used and abused by persons in the age groups subject to dementia. They produce a dreamy, relaxed state, and although they may impair concentration, they have no significant direct effect on memory. Narcotic drugs are often prescribed for severe pain. In general, their use for this purpose is entirely warranted and harmless. Withdrawal from narcotic drugs is uncomfortable but not nearly so dangerous as withdrawal from sedative drugs. There is also little danger of confusing withdrawal from narcotics with dementia.

Even so, there is one long-lasting though indirect effect of narcotic drugs that may contribute to brain dysfunction. Narcotic drugs decrease biological drives which may have serious consequences for elderly persons. Users may not eat enough or move about enough. They are likely to become severely constipated, dehydrated (starved of water) and malnourished. This generalized sluggishness may render a mildly impaired brain unable to compensate.

Stimulants

Here the danger actually seems to decrease with age. Caffeine is the most commonly used drug in this group. Some persons are unusually sensitive to the drug and become overly anxious and tremulous when taking it. Elderly people usually find this overarousal so disquieting that they voluntarily reduce their intake of coffee. Other stimulant drugs include amphetamine (Dexedrine and Methedrine are typical trade names), cocaine, and related drugs such as Ritalin. These drugs, too, seem to be rarely abused by elderly people. They are used mainly because they are prescribed by doctors in an attempt to improve mental functioning. The adverse publicity that surrounds them is mainly due to the epidemic of overuse of these drugs ("speed") by young people during the 1960s. There is a definite place for these drugs in improving the lot of the mildly impaired elderly person. Small dosages can bring about significant improvement in mental efficiency, concentration, and sense of well-being with little risk of abuse. However, stimulants are not a specific treatment for diseased brain tissue, and they must be used carefully.

Hallucinogenic Agents

This group includes marijuana, LSD, and several other "street" drugs. At present, few elderly persons probably use these drugs, but that may be changing with the generations. There is no information about their effects on the mental performance of elderly persons, let alone on dementia. On general pharmacologic grounds, we strongly recommend that these drugs be avoided. Even marijuana, which has a benign reputation and is even reputed to have beneficial effects (none have been proved), impairs brain function and is strongly suspected of having adverse long-term effects on young users. Moreover, "street" marijuana is commonly "laced" with other hallucinogenic drugs; phencyclidine (angel dust) is widely used today, but fashions change. These other drugs are capable of doing severe and lasting harm.

Prescribed Drugs

Other drugs taken by elderly persons are unlikely to be taken by choice; they are usually prescribed by physicians. Unfortunately, most drugs cause impairment of brain function in some circumstances, either directly or indirectly. Describing the effects of all of these drugs would be impractical and would contribute little useful information. The most frequent offenders are antidepressant drugs such as Tofranil and Elavil, drugs to lower blood pressure, drugs that calm or sedate the bowel, and drugs used for Parkinson's disease. The best rule is to suspect any drug that a person is taking of having an effect on that person's brain function. Be ever suspicious of pills, and be sure that any physician you consult about the possibility of dementing illness is aware of all drugs that have been prescribed for the patient and in what quantities and with what frequency they are actually taken.

4

Doctors: What They Do and How They Can Help

Those who must cope with dementing illness are likely to meet several specialists in medical practice, each offering particular expertise. These professionals are all highly trained, and most are fully competent. Understanding what these doctors do and how they go about doing it will give you a much better idea of what to expect from them and from the illness. This knowledge will help you plan, and it will also equip you to recognize superficial or incompetent medical practice should you encounter it.

Imagine yourself in the place of Harry's family doctor at the time his wife originally sought medical advice. First you set about defining the problem. You listen to the account of the events that brought Harry to you, and you pick out the main problem—loss of memory. Then you ask questions aimed at pinpointing the precise sort of memory loss (loss of recent memory), the duration of the loss (several weeks at least), and the type of onset and progression (insidious and gradual). While doing this, you mentally compile a list of all the diseases and processes that might produce the patterns the answers to your questions are revealing. Your list eventually includes most of the conditions we discussed in Chapters 2 and 3.

For example, you wonder whether the brain was injured. Therefore you ask, "Was there an accident? Unconsciousness? Paralysis?" and so on, until it is clear that injury is unlikely to have occurred. You inquire about alcohol and other drugs and ask Harry about depression: "How have your spirits been?" "Have you sometimes felt you would just as soon be dead?" "Have you ever thought of suicide?" "Has your weight changed?" In this way, you seek to eliminate possible causes and to focus on those diagnoses that are most likely. At this stage however, you keep all possible diagnoses in mind, no matter how unlikely some may seem. Given a problem as serious and difficult to assess as Harry's, many diagnoses will remain possible even after the most searching questions have been answered.

Sooner or later, as Harry's doctor, you probably decide that a complete examination is needed and proceed to ask questions that systematically probe for evidence of disordered function in every organ of the body. Headaches? . . . Blurred vision? . . . Joint pains? . . . Constipation? . . . and so on, through several dozen symptoms. A positive response to any of these questions leads to additional questions that explore further the system being reviewed. This procedure is known in medicine as the review of symptoms. You then do a complete physical examination, paying particular attention to any signs of disease of the brain or nerves. Finally, you order several laboratory examinations to screen for illnesses such as anemia, cancers of different kinds, infections such as syphilis and AIDS, and endocrine diseases.

Appendix A lists and briefly describes the component parts of a comprehensive set of laboratory tests useful when dementing illness is suspected. Physical findings, the historical information the doctor collects, or a positive result on one or another of these tests might send the investigation off in other directions. But the tests listed in Appendix A constitute a standard complete screening investigation. Illnesses capable of producing mental impairment are generally caught in the "net" of an examination by a competent physician backed by a clinical laboratory.

Though treatable illness rarely goes undetected, the consequences of not discovering it are extremely severe. Moreover, even after many possible diagnoses are eliminated, the doctor may still not have evidence that a specific illness *is* present and is causing the problem. Because of these uncertainties, the doctor often orders more elaborate diagnostic testing and asks consulting specialists to conduct other examinations and give their opinions.

Perhaps the process just described sounds as though it is routine practice that should proceed quickly and smoothly. But in the imperfect world in which we all live, physicians, not being infallible, may proceed hesitatingly. Like the rest of us, they are sometimes victims of false starts and blind alleys. In short, events most often move along at about the pace we observed in Harry's case.

Professional Specialists

The following medical specialists are likely to be concerned with dementing illness.

NEUROLOGIST A physician who deals mainly with diseases of the brain or nervous system, especially those that affect movement or consciousness. A neurologist or a psychiatrist is generally the primary physician in cases of dementia. These specialists have the most experience in investigating suspected dementing illness, and they usually provide ongoing medical care for those afflicted.

PSYCHIATRIST A physician who is especially concerned with diseases of the brain that produce disturbances in thinking or mood. The psychiatrist is also concerned with problematic behavior that may not be associated with diseases of the brain.

RADIOLOGIST A physician who uses radiation to diagnose or treat illness. In dementia, diagnosis is the only concern of the radiologist, and today the diagnostic procedures consist mainly of x-ray examinations. X-ray technology has become much more powerful and complex in the past decade, greatly augmenting the role of the radiologist.

PATHOLOGIST A physician who examines tissue to establish diagnoses. Pathologists also oversee most laboratory examinations of blood and other fluids. At an autopsy, the pathologist makes the final diagnosis. Neuropathologists specialize in the examination of tissue from the nervous system. A neuropathologist involved in a case of dementing illness is not likely to see the living patient, but only the neuropathologist or a general pathologist with extra qualifications in neuropathology is qualified to establish the final diagnosis.

To this listing should be added two nonmedically trained professionals who are likely to be involved in dealing with dementia.

PSYCHOLOGIST Psychologists are most important in the diagnostic effort. They administer and interpret psychological tests that provide essential diagnostic information about brain function. Confirmation that a dementing illness is or is not present is often provided by the results of psychological tests.

SOCIAL WORKER The social worker is the liaison among patients, families, and the many public and private agencies with which they may interact. A knowledgeable social worker can be immensely helpful to family members in dozens of practical ways. The staff of a hospital usually includes social workers, and often patients who become involved with nursing homes or public agencies are automatically assigned a social

worker. If this is not the practice in your area, ask your doctor
for a referral.

With the specialists come specialized diagnostic procedures. Those who may have dementing illnesses and their
families are almost always asked to consent to several examinations, and sometimes making that decision is not easy.
At the very least, responsible doctors should have the examinations well organized in order to minimize the time spent and
the confusion inherent in the process. Families should seek
assurance that steps have been taken to make the diagnostic
procedures as little disruptive of their lives as possible.

Remember that doctors seek certainty, and some may go
to undue lengths, ordering test after test until they come as
close as possible to achieving it. Of course being absolutely
certain would be wonderful, but at some point, the comfort
and well-being of the person undergoing the tests becomes
equally important (or even more so). Most doctors are sensitive to these considerations, but every situation is unique,
and the family must also exercise good judgment. Give the
doctor the benefit of any doubts, but at the same time, require
good, understandable reasons for everything asked of the
patient.

Finally, remember that throughout diagnosis and treatment, patients and families should ask themselves constantly,
"Are we getting the best available care?" The physician is
professionally obligated to provide the best possible care. Any
doctor who has any doubt about his or her ability to provide the
best care should request a consultation or refer the patient to
someone better prepared or better qualified. In addition,
patients and families always have the right to choose another
doctor. In the practical world, these matters are generally
settled via consultation. Families can always ask for a second
opinion from a doctor they choose before accepting the recommendation of their current doctor. Any doctor should accept
such a request in good grace, and nearly all do. You should
question the competence of any doctor who does otherwise. Do
not be hesitant or timid. When in doubt, act.

The following section describes the specialized tests and procedures that are most often advised and administered when dementia is suspected. These descriptions provide information that you may find useful when you ask questions of health care professionals.

Specialized Tests and Procedures

Psychological Testing

At present, the intellectual deficits of dementia, especially the loss of recent memory, can be most precisely estimated by means of psychological tests. Indeed, in the earliest stage of the dementing process, formal psychological testing may provide the only possible confirmation of deficits in memory formation. Because loss of recent memory is so characteristic of dementing illness, the tests that are used test mainly ability to learn new material. Failure to demonstrate memory impairments on psychological tests is strong evidence against the presence of dementia. As treatments are developed, psychological tests are also likely to be used to monitor their effects.

Some patients become extremely anxious when presented with psychological tests. However, a skilled and sensitive psychologist can usually overcome this problem, and many patients eventually come to enjoy the testing procedures. In general, psychological testing is harmless. Although repeat testing may be onerous because of the time required (often three to four hours), these tests provide useful measures of the progress of an illness. A few samples of test items appear in Appendix A. Appendix A also contains a scale that is used to assess roughly the progress of the dementing process over a period of time—on the order of six months. It can be administered in a few minutes, and it yields a numerical score.

The Electroencephalogram (EEG)

Often called the brain wave test, the electroencephalogram produces a recording of voltage patterns generated by the brain. These patterns are measured through electrodes applied to the scalp on each side of the head with a paste-like conductor. The procedure is painless and harmless, although the electrode paste in the hair is a little messy.

The brain characteristically produces a rhythm of 8 to 13 cycles per second from its mid and rearward parts. In the front, the rhythm is generally faster (14 to 22 cycles per second) and the change in voltage is smaller. By using several electrodes, it is possible to locate fairly precisely the voltage changes originating from a specific area of the brain. Normally, the two sides of the brain yield symmetrical recordings. In patients who suffer from dementia the recordings, though they are often not perfectly symmetrical, are generally not very unusual in this respect. Rather, the major change in dementia is a slowing of rhythm, and it tends not to occur until quite late in the course of dementing illness. Then the rhythm may slow to less than 8 cycles per second—often to 3 to 5 cycles per second. This change tends to be most prominent in areas of the brain that are involved with memory formation.

The value of the electroencephalogram is not that it can establish a diagnosis of primary dementia but rather that it can help the doctor eliminate from consideration other illnesses that may look like primary dementia. For example, if the normal symmetry of the recorded voltage is distorted, and especially if the asymmetry is fairly well localized, a tumor or stroke is more likely to be present than dementia.

An electroencephalogram may be ordered by any physician, although it is usually administered and read by a neurologist or sometimes a psychiatrist. Doctors may want to repeat the test several times through the course of the illness in order to follow its progress. This is entirely reasonable if taking the test does not overly upset the patient. In addition, the electroencephalogram may be needed in the investigation of seizures if these occur late in the course of the illness.

Cerebrospinal Fluid Examinations

During the first stages of investigating a dementing illness, doctors obtain a sample of cerebrospinal fluid. Some tests to eliminate important diseases from consideration can be performed in no other way. For example, syphilis, a disease that is by no means rare, may be present in the brain and reveal itself in cerebrospinal fluid even though the conventional tests on blood are negative. And there are several other diseases that manifest themselves most clearly in cerebrospinal fluid.

Obtaining cerebrospinal fluid may sound dangerous, but it is actually a routine procedure that any doctor can perform. The pain and discomfort are moderate—hardly more than the prick of a needle. Because the needle enters the cavity containing the fluid at a point several inches below the end of the spinal cord itself, there is no possibility of paralysis because of injury to the spine. Indeed, the procedure has only one fairly common side effect: a throbbing headache that may last for a few hours. Fortunately, severe headaches not only are rare but can be easily treated.

X-Rays and the CAT Scan

Conventional x-ray examinations are of limited value in investigating dementia because they can provide only an image of the skull, not the brain. They are used instead as a crude screen to reveal other pathological processes that might mimic dementia. In recent years, however, several new techniques have been developed that yield images of brain tissue itself. These advances have been truly revolutionary. Their contribution to diagnosis and research has hardly begun to be realized. Among these new techniques, computerized axial tomography (the CAT scan) is the most important when dementia is suspected. The CAT scan can outline the brain, including both surface and ventricles. Moreover, it can do this in simulated "slices" so that the brain can be visualized at several levels. For example, an image of the brain can be produced on a horizontal plane (a

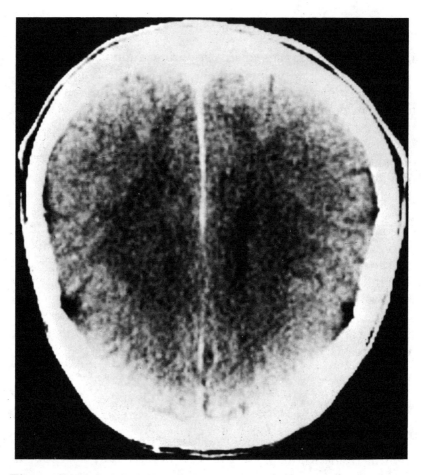

Figure 3a Results of CAT scans. The brain above is normal. *Courtesy of Dr. Larry Gold.*

plane parallel to the floor) at the level of the eyebrows. Figure 3 shows two typical slices.

   This amazing technology has replaced several older procedures, including pneumoencephalography, which had been particularly important in investigating possible dementia. That procedure, which produced severe side effects, is now

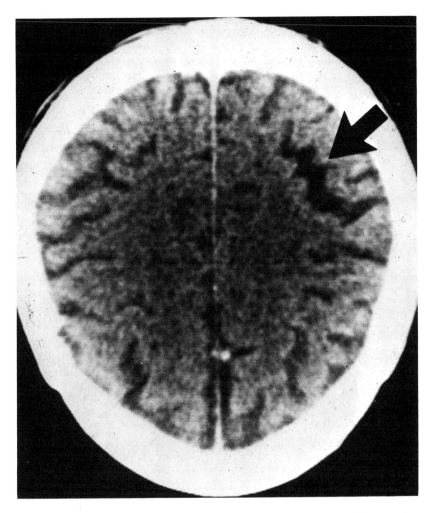

Figure 3b Results of CAT scans. The brain above is shrunken consistent with a progressive dementia. The arrow indicates a crevice on the surface of the brain (sulci), which widens because the brain itself shrinks. *Courtesy of Dr. Larry Gold.*

happily obsolete. The CAT scan enables us actually to see evidence of multiple small injuries such as minor strokes or tumors, which can produce an outcome much like dementia. It can also reveal low-pressure hydrocephalus. For these purposes the CAT scan is unique and irreplaceable. However, it is only fairly late in the course of dementia that the telltale shrinkage of the brain that betrays dementia becomes unmistakable on the CAT scan. Therefore, a CAT scan may not provide proof that an early dementia is present. With age, some symmetrical shrinkage of the brain occurs even in mentally intact normal persons, whereas little shrinkage may be present in the early stages of dementia. Thus there is so much overlap between CAT scans from normal persons and from those with early dementia that definitive diagnosis on the basis of a CAT scan is not usually possible. Its crucial contribution is the elimination of other causes of dementia.

Brain Biopsy

It is possible surgically to remove a small sample of brain tissue through a hole made in the skull, and a pathologist can often use this tissue to make a conclusive diagnosis. Obtaining a piece of tissue for diagnostic purposes is known in medicine as performing a biopsy. The surgery need not affect brain function in any measurable way, because the amount of brain tissue removed is small and it is removed from a "silent" area—a part of the brain that has no specific function.

Despite its lack of measurable effect on the brain, however, biopsy has little if any place in the current management of dementing illness. Biopsy necessitates general anesthesia and that entails a significant risk. Entry through the skull is not a benign procedure, and it may produce discomfort throughout the postoperative period and into convalescence. These deterrents would matter little if the procedure could make any practical difference in outcome, but it cannot. In all except the rarest cases, having a correct diagnosis during life does not affect treatment. Moreover, early in the course of the illness, the changes in brain tissue are not so widespread that they are certain to appear in a small sample of tissue. Consequently, accurate diagnosis might not be possible even with a biopsy.

In the future, effective treatments for one or more of the primary dementing illnesses may well appear, and then the opportunity to determine which treatment to apply may justify the patient's undergoing the trauma of brain biopsy in order to get an exact diagnosis. By then we may also have discovered methods of examining tissue that are more effective than those the microscope now provides. But these developments are still in the future. For now, only exceptional circumstances provide sufficient justification for inflicting the risk and discomfort of surgery on persons with dementia. A doctor who suggests biopsy should be able to explain the need for it to the full satisfaction of family members. A diagnosis is extremely important, but in all but the rarest circumstances, pathological examination can wait until the autopsy.

The Autopsy

The importance of a pathological examination of brain tissue obtained by autopsy cannot be overstated. It is at present the only way in which a conclusive diagnosis can be established, and it is likely to remain so well into the future. Without an examination of brain tissue, the best diagnosis is still only a clinical opinion, and for the reasons listed below, that is just not reliable enough for most serious purposes.

Autopsy is often difficult to contemplate or discuss. To the professional, the autopsy is no more than surgery performed after death. But nonprofessionals who do not share that perspective may not be able to concentrate on dispassionate explanations, especially when recently bereaved. Even when the survivors understand the importance of accurate diagnosis, giving permission to obtain it through autopsy may be difficult. Relatives may imagine that disfigurement, disrespectful handling of tissue, and mutilation are likely to result. (These fears are unfounded.) For some, religious beliefs may forbid authorizing the procedure. Often relatives just want to see a quick end of the disease process and say something like "He has suffered enough already." Finally, there is the question

"What good is an autopsy going to do him(or her)?" The answer, of course, is "none at all," but for survivors, having an accurate diagnosis is extremely important. Let's review the reasons why.

1. As treatments are developed, each will probably be effective only for one specific illness. Because the probability is so high that anyone who develops a dementing illness has the same illness as any similarly affected family member, being certain what dementing illness that other family member had enables the new patient's doctor to make a presumptive diagnosis quickly and begin treatment without delay. This may save a great deal of time and thereby prevent the destruction of brain tissue. It may also make it unnecessary to "try out" treatments that might be uncomfortable or dangerous and would prove ineffective. These benefits extend indefinitely. Tissue samples and slides are often preserved by pathologists. Thus making them available for future examinations, which may well include new diagnostic procedures that can be applied in the future.

2. The various dementing illnesses carry different genetic risks and have different natural histories. Knowing which illness threatens the family will help family members plan realistically.

3. Brain tissue is essential to many of the research programs that are most likely to bring to light the basic biochemical, physiologic, and pharmacologic properties of the progressive dementias. Remember that no animal develops a condition precisely analogous to the neuropathology of dementia of the Alzheimer type (DAT). It is hard to say even that an animal *can* develop dementia. At this time, tissue is needed most from two sources: persons without brain disease to serve as controls, and persons with DAT in whom the course of the disease has been especially well documented or

whose family members are especially well known. The need for control tissue is particularly critical.

The questions families seem to ask most often about autopsies are these:

1. "Who can give permission for an autopsy?" In order of their legal standing, the following relatives can give permission: spouse, adult son or daughter, parent, and adult sibling. Among relatives, the one with the highest legal standing who is available and competent must agree. That is, if a spouse is living, competent, and available, that spouse must agree in order for an autopsy to be preformed. If such a spouse withholds permission, no other relative or combination of relatives can override his or her decision. However, a legally appointed guardian or a judge who has jurisdiction can order an autopsy.

2. "To whom should the permission be given?" In nearly all cases, the physician who last attended the deceased is in a position to arrange for the autopsy. Assistance may also be available from the Alzheimer's Association, a local medical association, or a local pathologist. The Alzheimer's Association has created a nationwide autopsy assistance network of qualified volunteers to assist families. Appendix B contains the address of the national Alzheimer's Association and the 800 number to call for referral to the nearest autopsy representative. Local Alzheimer's Association chapters are listed in telephone directories. There are similar lay organizations concerned with Huntington's disease and hereditary ataxias, which, though not strictly dementias, are a related group of brain diseases. Appendix C lists contacts for other organizations devoted to Alzheimer's and related disorders.

3. "Can we have an open casket if an autopsy is done?" Of course. There is no disfigurement at all. The only

visible sign is a cut in the skin at the back of the neck and that can be seen only on close inspection.

4. "Can we learn what was found?" Yes. It takes at least six weeks to process tissue, examine it, and prepare a report. That report is available to immediate relatives, and most doctors are glad to explain it in detail. Diagnoses are entered on death certificates at the time of death. If the autopsy reveals a different cause, the death certificate should be amended. (Make sure that this is done.)

5. "Should the entire body be studied?" In general, yes, especially when there is any doubt about the cause of death. However, only brain tissue is needed to establish a specific diagnosis from among the progressive dementias.

These are the major issues families consider. Together with conscience and sensitivity, they can guide families to sensible decisions.

CHAPTER 5

Causes of Primary Dementia: Fact and Fiction

We do not know what causes primary dementia. Even to speak of a single cause is misleading, because dementia is the result of a complicated sequence of events that involves many contributing factors. Chronic illnesses such as arthritis, diabetes, and cancer have taught medical science many painful lessons: One is that simple causes are illusory.

In this chapter, we shall take up the factors known to contribute to dementia or strongly suspected of doing so. Each should be thought of not as a cause in itself, but rather as another piece of the puzzle. To the caregiver or relative of someone who suffers from a dementing illness this description of the limits of knowledge is likely to be disheartening. But these limits are expanding at rates that have few precedents in science.

Genetic Factors

Genes are the single causal factor that has been convincingly demonstrated to be at work in most dementing illnesses. Viral infection is the only other cause generally accepted by scientists, but viruses and genes are intimately linked. In fact, genes provide a biological framework around which all other causal factors can be organized. However, these causal chains will certainly not be simple structures to untangle: Not a single link is yet thoroughly understood. To begin with, the action of genes cannot be understood except in relation to the environment in which they operate. Genes basically respond to moment-to-moment changes in that environment. Moreover, diseases with effects as broad as the dementias surely involve a large proportion of the genes of the body in one way or another. And most fairly common diseases, such as dementia of the Alzheimer type (DAT) probably have several different forms, each one associated with different genes or combinations of genes.

We will first describe the basic inheritance of dementing illness as established by family and pedigree studies. Then we will touch on one of the most active and productive areas in all of science, the molecular mechanisms of gene action, where profound change is in the wind. Recent advances in basic biological science have made it possible to determine the structure of all human genes and to map their positions relative to one another. This great revolution is as far-reaching as any in the history of our species. For those concerned with dementia, it is especially significant.

Huntington's Disease

Huntington's disease provides the most straightforward introduction to genetic factors in dementia. Its inheritance seems simple, because almost exactly 50 percent of the first-degree relatives (the parents, siblings, and children) of an affected person are themselves affected. First-degree relatives share an average of 50 percent of their genes. This 50 percent constitutes a genetic ratio, the one associated with a dominant gene. However, this seemingly simple picture is complicated by several factors. Thus we will use Huntington's disease to introduce general properties of genetics applied to dementia.

One such general property is this: We cannot tell from the information now available just how many different diseases appear to us as the single illness we know as Huntington's disease. Separate variants of the disease have not been identified, yet we must strongly suspect that such variants exist. So many examples of the splitting of what was thought to be one disease into two, or three, or more have been found that no one with experience in medical genetics would be surprised to learn that variants of Huntington's disease had been likewise "teased apart." It is likely that progress in understanding dementing illnesses will proceed stepwise. Each step will mark a discovery involving one among several forms of each disease, and an approach that is effective in treating one variant may not benefit another.

As in other progressive dementias, the manifestations of Huntington's disease can vary widely. It can begin in infancy or in extreme old age. It may emerge as a fulminating (explosive) illness or as an indolent, barely progressing one. A peculiar involuntary writhing movement usually marks the disease, but some cases feature muscular rigidity, and in others there is no apparent involvement of muscles at all. Highly regarded physicians have wrongly diagnosed cases of the latter kind as DAT. Some persons known to possess the gene for Huntington's disease have lived into their seventies and eighties without exhibiting signs of the illness. (Presumably they would have shown signs eventually, but they did not live long enough.) All of these types of variability must be attributed to genes that modify the action of the gene that causes the disease, to environmental factors, or to some combination of genes and environment. Such complicated causal networks are the general rule in chronic disease.

Huntington's disease also illustrates the effect of age at onset on the probability that a given relative of an affected person will develop the same disease. For example, we know that half of the children of a person who has Huntington's disease will become affected. We also know that the average age at onset of the illness is about 40; that is, half of the cases develop before that age and half after. Now, what is the "remaining risk" to the 40-year-old son or daughter of an affected person? It started as 0.5 (or one-half) but now it must be less because some—40 years—of the period for which the individual is at risk has been lived through without sign of disease. But just how much less? This question comes up again and again in practice. Sadly, the common-sense answer is not the correct one. It seems at first that if the initial risk was 1/2 and if half of the cases have developed by about age 40, then the risk should be reduced by half and become 1/4 (or one in every four). However, this solution overlooks the fact that the sibling at risk in our example may have been one of the 50 percent who did not inherit the gene at birth.

The probabilities are complicated to describe but easy to see. Figure 4 is a diagram of the probabilities. It shows that 50 percent of the children of a person affected with Huntington's disease will have the gene. Half of that 50 percent of the children who got the gene at birth, or 25 percent of all the children, will develop the disease by age 40. Of course, the 50 percent of children who did not get the gene will not develop the disease at all. As the legend that accompanies Figure 4 explains, those who will develop the disease after age 40 constitute one-third of all of those who remain well at age 40. Therefore, the actual remaining risk is 0.33, not 0.25, or one chance in three rather than one chance in four.

Grasping this concept will probably take a little study of Figure 4, but some acquaintance with these calculations is fundamental to understanding genetic risks and discussing them with health-care professionals. The basic data you need to work with include the distribution of observed ages at onset of illness. Table 6 gives this information for

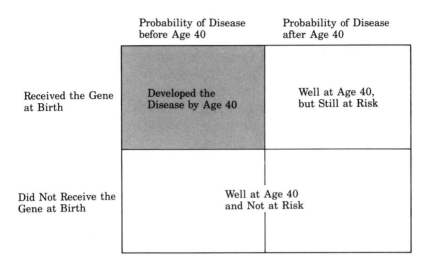

	Probability of Disease before Age 40	Probability of Disease after Age 40
Received the Gene at Birth	Developed the Disease by Age 40	Well at Age 40, but Still at Risk
Did Not Receive the Gene at Birth	Well at Age 40 and Not at Risk	

Figure 4 Diagrammatic representation of the remaining risk for a first-degree relative of a known victim of Huntington's disease. The large rectangle (as a whole) represents the total probability of getting Huntington's disease for the newborn child of a person who has the gene for Huntington's disease. Half of such children (here represented as the top two smaller rectangles) will have received the gene (they are called carriers). The other half of the children inherited normal genes from their parents and will remain normal. By age 40, half of those who have the gene will have developed the disease. The shaded area represents these individuals, and the remaining three areas represent all those who, whatever their genetic makeup, have not developed Huntington's disease by age 40. Of course, those who did not get the gene at birth, have no risk of ever developing the disease. Those still at risk,then represented by the upper right quadrant, constitute one-third of those who are well at age 40. Therefore, the remaining risk for those who are well at age 40 is one-third, or 0.33.

Huntington's disease. The algebra you need to use these distributions (and similar distributions for other diseases) may look formidable at first, but it is really quite simple. Appendix D contains the formula and several worked-out examples.

Table 6 Age at Onset of Huntigton's Disease*

Age at onset (years)	Percent with onset	Cumulative percent
–10	0.1	0.1
11–15	0.7	0.8
16–20	1.4	2.2
21–25	3.2	5.4
26–30	7.6	13.0
31–35	8.9	21.9
36–40	13.4	35.3
41–45	16.4	51.7
46–50	19.8	71.5
51–55	14.0	85.5
56–60	9.6	95.1
61–65	3.5	98.6
66–70	1.1	99.7
71–	0.3	100.0

*Lifetime empirical risk for first-degree relatives is estimated as 0.5

DAT

Predicting the remaining risk of developing DAT is more difficult than for Huntington's disease. Figure 5 illustrates the basic data. The lines in the graph represent cumulative risks at the indicated ages for relatives of a persons with DAT. For example, the risk to siblings up to age 75 is about 7 percent. This risk is the sum of the risks to age 65 (about 1 percent), between age 66 and 70 (about 2.5 percent), and between age 71 and age 75 (about 3.5 percent). The lines are reasonably straight, which means that the added risk during each age interval is fairly constant—3 to 4 percent. There are no estimates available for children, because no families have been studied long enough for children to grow up and become affected. However, children probably run about the same risk as siblings. Second-degree relatives (for example, uncles, aunts,

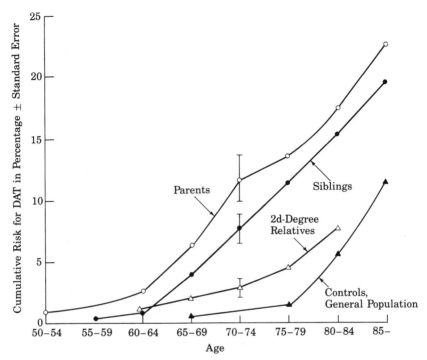

Figure 5 Cumulative age-specific risk of developing dementia of the Alzheimer type (DAT) for parents, siblings, second-degree relatives, and the general population.

and grandchildren) have a considerably reduced risk, as genetic theory predicts, and are affected only in high-risk families, as will be described below. The risks for third-degree relatives (first cousins) merge with those for the general population.

It is important to underscore that the risks graphed in Figure 5 are age-specific; they are the risks of becoming affected *by any specified age.* Usually, only overall percentage risks are cited—for example, 50 percent for a first-degree relative of a person with Huntington's disease. But clearly, in the case of DAT, the practical impact of a given risk differs considerably for persons of age 50, say, and age 80. When data are available, age-specific risks are much more informative than overall risks.

As depicted by the rightmost line in Figure 5, at older ages DAT begins to occur among members of the general population, and it eventually affects some 20 to 30 percent of those of us who live long enough. Viewed from this perspective, the main effect of having a first-degree relative with DAT is a greater risk of developing the disease earlier in life than someone without such a relative. This difference in age can be roughly estimated from Figure 5. Place a ruler parallel to the x-axis of the graph (the x-axis is the bottom horizontal line) at the 5 percent point of the y-axis. You will see that the ruler crosses the Siblings line at about age 66 and crosses the General Population line at about age 80, a difference of fourteen years.

The risks shown in Figure 5 are not really large compared to many others inherent in life. Most relatives of a person with DAT can simply ignore them as being of no real significance. However, families wherein severe disease has occurred face appreciably greater risks. Among the most straightforward ways to identify such families is to consider age at onset and proportion of relatives affected. Early onset suggests increased severity; and the larger the proportion of relatives affected, the greater the severity. In pooled data from a large number of families, parents are the relatives who can most conveniently be used to estimate the proportion of relatives affected, because everyone has only two biological parents, whereas the numbers of siblings and children vary widely. Also, parents are always older than their children and have therefore been exposed to the age-related risks experienced by any other first-degree relative. For individuals, parents are still the best overall guide, but age at onset is also helpful when estimating risks. Figure 6 depicts the risks for the siblings of persons with DAT whose illness began either before or after age 70 and, in the case of onset before age 70, whose parent either was or was not affected. The risks for relatives of a victim of DAT whose onset occurred at age 70 or older is hardly different from the risk for members of the general population (see Figure 5). The magnitude of the risk increases for relatives who developed the

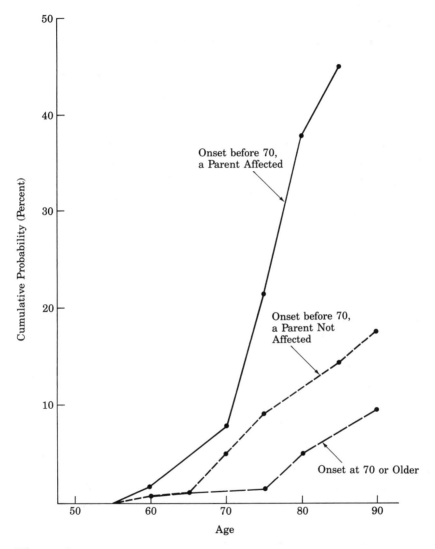

Figure 6 Cumulative age-specific risks to siblings of persons who developed dementia of the Alzheimer type (DAT) at age 70 or older and to siblings of persons who developed DAT before age 70 and who had or did not have an affected parent.

disease before age 70. For persons who had both a relative with onset before 70, and an affected parent, the risk becomes much more substantial, reaching 45 percent by age 70. Happily, there are few such families. Many more families at risk are in the lowest-risk groups, and in two-thirds of all families that include one affected person no one else is affected at all.

These estimates may have to be modified in the light of more recent research. Although reported empirical risks to relatives have been remarkably consistent among studies for persons and families averaging more youthful onset of illness (up to age 70), newer results suggest that the overall risk for first-degree relatives of affected persons of even late-onset families may approach 50 percent. These studies assessed illness in advanced age ranges for which data either were not available to earlier investigators or were discounted by them. There are two reasons for such discounting. It is very difficult to have confidence in the diagnosis of dementing illness in elderly persons because they so often have chronic diseases of the heart or other organs that might affect brain functioning. And the risk of DAT increases sharply in the general population at advanced ages, making it hard to attribute cases observed in families under investigation to specific inherited genes. These issues cannot be resolved except through new research. In the meantime, we recommend basing estimates of risk on Figures 5 and 6, and on Table 7, which contains a distribution of ages at onset.

One source of confusion about risk is that families seem to have such variable proportions of affected members; some have several, others none. The answer is that sheer luck plays a large part in human affairs. This good or bad fortune has its basis in simple probability, which we can illustrate by briefly exploring a sample problem. Suppose that the risk for development of illness is 20 percent (or one chance in five) for the children of a person with a given disease and that we seek the probabilities for a family with four children. For each birth, we draw a marble out of an urn containing one red marble and four white ones, where the red marble designates an individual destined to develop the disease. Then the probability of getting four

Table 7 Age at Onset for Dementia of the Alzheimer Type*

Age at onset (years)	Percent with onset	Cumulative percent
–44	2	2
45–49	3	5
50–54	5	10
55–59	7	17
60–64	14	31
65–69	19	50
70–74	17	67
75–79	16	83
80–84	12	95
85–	5	100

*Lifetime empirical risk for first-degree relatives is estimated as 0.30. But risks are age-specific and vary with family type. If possible, use risks estimated from Figures 5 and 6 in Chapter 5.

white marbles in four draws, corresponding to none affected, is 41 percent; the probability of one being affected is also 41 percent; that of two being affected is 15 percent; of three, 3 percent; and of four, 0.1 percent (the total slightly exceeds 100 percent because of rounding). Thus 41 percent of all the genetically at-risk groups of four siblings are never recognized because no member develops the disease, whereas, simply by the (bad) luck of the draw, other families seem to be at especially high risk. Similar calculations can be made for families of any size. Genetic analyses allow for such chance events, but they can mislead those who are trying to apply common sense to their family's experience.

Pick's Disease

Pick's disease is rarer than Huntington's disease and much rarer than DAT. It is important to remember that Pick's and

DAT occur in different age ranges. As we have seen, DAT may, in extremely rare cases, begin in the third decade of life. By the fifth decade, it is still a rare disease, but then the frequency of its onset increases steadily throughout the remaining human life span.

Huntington's and Pick's diseases exhibit quite different patterns of occurrence than that of DAT. Instead of increasing steadily, the numbers of new cases of both of these diseases rise to a peak in the middle years of life and then decrease. The distributions of ages at onset are fairly symmetrical around means. This is the general experience with disease: for example, rheumatoid arthritis, schizophrenia, and multiple sclerosis exhibit this sort of pattern, and there is therefore a possibility of outliving the risk for these diseases. In contrast, the frequency of DAT increases throughout the life span. In this

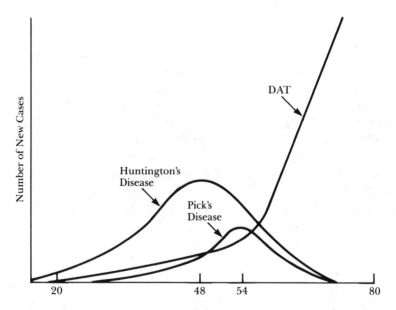

Figure 7 Schematic distributions of age at onset of DAT, Huntington's disease, and Pick's disease.

Table 8 Age at Onset for Pick's Disease*

Age at onset, (years)	Percent falling ill	Cumulative percent
–39	7	7
40–49	13	20
50–59	38	58
60–69	28	86
70–	14	100

*Lifetime empirical risk for first-degree relatives is estimated as 0.25.

it is more like other highly age-related conditions such as occlusive arterial disease and loss of functioning kidney cells. These relationships are illustrated in Figure 7.

The frequency of onset of Pick's disease increases more rapidly than that of DAT through about age 54. Even at maximum frequency, it remains a rare disease. Then its frequency of onset decreases, and new cases beginning over age 75 are rare. The average survival after onset is seven to eight years—somewhat shorter than the average survival of persons with DAT with onsets in the same age ranges. Earlier onset in Pick's disease, as in DAT, is likely to be associated with a shorter course and with greater severity.

The risk that relatives run is not so well defined for Pick's disease as for DAT. Studies based on just a few families suggest lifetime risks of 25 percent for parents and of 20 percent for siblings. Age-specific risks and a distrubution of onset ages for Pick's disease are presented in Table 8. No risk for children has been directly determined. Here again, the risk for siblings (20 percent) would be the best estimate.

Molecular Genetics

Now that we have examined how applying genetic principles can help us predict the risk that relatives of a person affected with certain dementing illnesses will develop the same disease, let us briefly examine the molecular mechanisms of gene action associated with the diseases that produce dementia.

Over the past decade, astounding progress has been made in the study of molecular genetics—the molecular mechanisms associated with disease. Moreover, it appears ever more likely that this is the level at which treatment will be focused. Huntington's disease, DAT, and Gerstmann–Sträusseler syndrome are coming to be understood at the molecular level. In addition, scientists are investigating the molecular bases of some viral diseases that produce dementia. Molecular genetics is now leading the way toward comprehensive understanding of disease, including dementia. However, knowledge has accumulated so fast that the general level of basic education, including that of physicians, is not adequate to keep pace. Indeed, modern genetics is leading a revolution with practical and philosophical implications as profound as any in the history of our species. The next pages present the essential concepts underlying this revolution. It is neither a comprehensive account nor, we fear, easy reading. But our overview will at least cover the major developments in dementia research.

One of the substances within our bodies is deoxyribonucleic acid, or DNA. The information our cells need to carry on the processes of life is contained in DNA in the form of a code: the genetic code. The coding components of DNA are four relatively small molecules, the nucleic acids, which are arranged in long strands and separated into packages called chromosomes. Normally, there are 46 chromosomes in each of our cells, 23 of which we inherit from our mother and 23 from our father. The order in which the four organic bases line up in DNA strands is also inherited from our parents: Half are arranged in sequences transmitted from our mothers, half in sequences transmitted from our fathers. Think of the bases as beads of four different colors strung on 46 immensely long strings. The strings are so long because, with exceptions unimportant for our purposes, each cell of our body contains about 6,000,000,000 (six billion) nucleic acids.

DNA has several functions. As is well known, it can make exact copies of itself, thereby permitting reproduction. DNA also has two basic functions pertinent to disease. First, the order of bases (the beads) in DNA determines the structure of our proteins. Second, DNA participates in regulating the amount of specific proteins produced at any given moment throughout life. Together, differences in protein structure and differences in regulation account for the range of biological diversity that our species exhibits. This diversity includes disease.

A special property of DNA makes possible most of the applications of "high tech" biology to clinical medicine. This property is the effectively invariant pairing of the bases that make up the coding segment of DNA. The four coding bases are adenine, cytosine, guanine, and thymine, they are usually designated by their initials, A, C, G, and T. (Substitute colors such as *A*zure, *C*rimson, *G*reen, and *T*eal if you wish) In nature and in the laboratory, A pairs with T, and C pairs with G. Thus a sequence of bases, say A-A-T-C-C, for example, will anneal with T-T-A-G-G rapidly, and with near perfect fidelity to form a double strand. Because of this property, a single strand of DNA can be used as a probe to seek its complementary strand. This pairing forms the basis for much of molecular genetics and explains the origin of the term *recombinant DNA*.

Structure of Proteins

Some DNA segments code for specific amino acids to be linked together to form proteins. A sequence of three nucleic acids specifies one amino acid out of the 20 that make up our proteins. As examples, A-C-G codes for the amino acid threonine, and T-T-T codes for phenylalanine. A segment of DNA some several thousand nucleic acids long contains the information needed to make one chain of amino acids. Such a chain may itself constitute a complete protein, but most are processed after manufacture, being joined to other chains, for example, to make a more complex protein.

Proteins, in their turn, are the stuff of life—its bricks, mortar, and tools. DNA supplies the information necessary for life; proteins organize and perform life's work. It may be helpful to think of proteins as divided into two types. One type makes up the structure of the body. These structural proteins not only form our physical matrix, but also manufacture nonprotein molecules such as hormones and neurotransmitters. Many structural proteins incorporate, for use or transport, small molecules such as minerals, fats, sugars, and vitamins. The second type consists of regulatory proteins. They are also coded for by DNA segments, and they interact with DNA that codes for structural proteins in such a way as to increase or decrease production of specific structural proteins. The mechanism through which this is accomplished will be outlined later. For now, the important point is that structural and regulatory proteins together constitute the organizing framework of the body.

If, through a chance event (a mutation), one nucleic acid is substituted for another in a DNA segment, say C for the second G in G-G-C making G-C-C, then the amino acid alanine is substituted for glycine in the protein coded for by that DNA segment. Such substitution is one type of mutation, the simplest to describe. Others include the deletion or the addition of nucleic acids. Mutations occur at random. What effect one will have depends on where it occurs. A difference in protein structure that results from mutation may be entirely without practical effect on life; or it may alter the product of that segment just enough to make it slightly less efficient or more efficient, or enough to predispose to disease. In the forgoing example, the substitution of alanine for glycine in a specific protein is associated with phenylketonuria, a disease that produces profound mental retardation. It is no surprise in view of what we are learning about the complexity of diseases, that 12 other alterations in the same protein, caused by different mutations, are known to produce phenylketonuria. Also typically, the effective treatment is elimination of phenylalanine from the diet—an adjustment of the environment. Without the environmental codeterminant, there is no disease.

Regulation of Protein Production

DNA determines the structure of proteins but it also acts in conjunction with other molecules to control the amounts of structural protein produced by specific DNA segments. This control is the response of individual cells to their environment: Ultimately, it is the mechanism through which we respond to our external environments. Regulatory proteins are the essential control elements, but nonprotein molecules such as hormones also regulate genes. Because these nonprotein molecules are themselves made or organized by proteins, it is apparent that DNA itself contains the information needed for its own regulation. Exactly how this is done mechanically is not known in detail, but the processes are rapidly being unraveled by research. Broadly speaking, some DNA segments are configured in such a way as to provide sites for the attachment of regulatory molecules. Such unions can decrease or increase the decoding of specific DNA segments and hence lessen or augment production of particular products. The effects are finely graded across a range from complete blocking of production to massive increases. Like structural sites, regulatory sites on DNA are also subject to mutation with consequent change in functional capacity.

The substances that unite with DNA are, then, the direct or indirect products of other DNA segments. Some may be produced in response to "housekeeping" demands, such as those imposed by internal timing or "clock" mechanisms. But many regulatory substances are produced in response to changes in the external environment. DNA is constantly fine-tuning our responses to ongoing change in external environments, and these responses include storing memories in the brain and in the immune system.

DNA and Disease

The first step in successful searches for the causes of genetic disease is to locate approximately disease-associated DNA segments on specific chromosomes. This localization is called linkage: The disease-associated segment is "linked" to a specific chromosome. The establishment of linkage makes it possible to "close in on" those DNA segments progressively by locating markers on either side of them until, eventually, they are isolated. The next step is to determine the base sequence of that DNA segment. Working from the genetic code, investigators can infer the structure of any protein produced by that segment.

If all or part of the segment is regulatory and codes for no protein, the next steps are not so clear-cut. Considerable trial-and-error research may be needed, but the technology now available will make it possible ultimately to define the relevant genetic mechanisms. This entails determining (1) to what environmental factors the regulatory mechanism responds and (2) what product it regulates in what direction (toward more or less of it) in response to change in that environment.

After this work is completed, DNA segments associated with disease, the equivalent normal segments, and the products of each can be directly compared. Finally, a way to bypass or neutralize the damage done by the defective segment is sought in order to provide effective treatments. This process has not yet been completed for any illness, but it is well along in some cases (such as cystic fibrosis), and there is little doubt that dementing illness can be approached in the same way.

Molecular Genetics of DAT

Family studies demonstrated that genetic transmission plays a part in DAT, so following the general plan just outlined, the DNA segments involved were urgently sought. An important byproduct of this research was the rediscovery of the relationship between Alzheimer's disease and Down's syndrome. All persons with Down's syndrome have been found, upon autopsy, to have had in their brain tissues the plaques and tangles characteristic of Alzheimer's disease. This critical clue pointed researchers toward the chromosome, chromosome 21, that is aberrant in Down's syndrome. These developments set the stage for the advent of molecular genetics in DAT.

Molecular investigations of DAT then followed two pathways. One flowed with exemplary logic from the pathology depicted in Figure 1 (in Chapter 2). Senile plaques have a core composed of amyloid, a small protein fragment. The amino acid sequence of amyloid was worked out and this made it possible to decipher the DNA sequence that coded for it. That DNA sequence was found to anneal to DNA from chromosome 21.

Those who followed the other pathway began with the family studies. They sought evidence of genetic linkage by using a basic tool of molecular genetics, the fragment-length polymorphism. Fragment-length polymorphisms are fragments of DNA that vary in length from individual to individual and they are the best available landmarks identifying DNA segments. The fragments are produced by exposing DNA to endonucleases, which are enzymes present in bacteria to protect against invasion by foreign DNA. (Bacteria are subject to infection too.) Each such enzyme—several dozen are known—splits DNA at a specific point identified by a sequence of six (or so) bases. Every time the enzyme recognizes its sequence, it cuts the DNA. When DNA from an individual is exposed to any one of the enzymes, it is split into millions of fragments. Because of mutations, every individual differs from every other individual in the number of DNA sequences that a particular enzyme recognizes and cuts (excepting only identical twins). For example, say a certain enzyme recognizes T-G-G-T-A, and cuts the DNA chain in response to that sequence. If any of the nucleic acids is changed (say A is changed to T yielding T-G-G-T-T), the cut will not be made. The result is that each of us is identified by the length of the fragments produced. Because variation in DNA produces the different lengths, the polymorphism (literally, "many shapes") is inherited according to known genetic laws and can be traced from generation to generation. However, too many fragments are produced by treatment of all of an individual's DNA to be efficiently managed by current techniques. Therefore, practical use of the method depends on localizing DNA segment associated with a

trait of interest to an area no greater than one chromosome—
that is, establishing linkage. (In the near future, genetic "maps"
locating polymorphic markers very close to one another across
all chromosomes will be available and will make feasible
screening searches for genes associated with any trait.)

As described earlier, fragment-length polymorphisms
mark chromosomes, thus making it possible to identify those
those that carry disease-associated genes. Suppose that in a
given family, all or nearly all persons affected by DAT have a
DNA fragment of a particular length whereas all or nearly all
unaffected persons in the families have a longer (or shorter)
fragment from the same area of a chromosome. This association
between DAT and fragment length, if constant within families,
would link the disease to a particular DNA segment.

Although large families of suitable composition in which
the diagnosis of DAT has been reasonably established are rare,
linkage between disease and DNA fragments from chromosome
21 has been confirmed by several research groups. As soon as
this linkage was demonstrated, linkage was also sought between the DAT segment and the amyloid segments. Indeed, it
was thought possible that the amyloid segment itself caused
the disease. It was a surprise, though a mild one, when the
amyloid segment of chromosome 21 was demonstrated to be
entirely independent of the DAT segment. Both a DAT segment
and an amyloid segment are on human chromosome 21, but
they are a long way apart.

More recently, two research groups have been unable to
demonstrate linkage of DAT to chromosome 21, and one found
linkage to chromosome 19. Such divergence should be expected.
Some of it will surely prove to be due to different DNA segments, producing the same end result: DAT. Some divergence
will probably also prove to be due to the fact that the statistical
calculations involved are extremely sensitive to diagnostic
error. Today, linkage of DAT to chromosome 21 can be regarded
as established in some families, but in other families the
disease is associated with other chromosomes. But that is not
the important conclusion. Molecular studies have demonstrated that the tools are in hand that will eventually isolate

the DNA segments associated with DAT. The question is not whether this will be done, but rather how soon.

Meanwhile, there is more to be gleaned from the relationship between DAT and Down's syndrome, a condition due to the presence in every cell of three instead of the normal two copies of chromosome 21. While Down's syndrome produces brain changes identical to those produced by DAT, the DNA possessed by persons with Down's syndrome must be normal in structure. All cases of Down's syndrome could hardly possess the same mutant DNA associated with Alzheimer's disease in persons with the normal two copies of chromosome 21. It follows that the pathology of Down's syndrome is associated with the 50 percent excess of DNA that is present because of the extra copy of chromosome 21 present in Down's syndrome. It is known that the 50 percent excess DNA produces roughly 50 percent excess product and that excess product must be associated with the pathology of Down's syndrome including the brain changes. DAT could also be associated with an excess of chromosome 21 product due to a mutation resulting in faulty regulation of a group of chromosome 21 genes, perhaps including the amyloid gene. Many examples of this sort of regulation are known in nature. The Down's relationship has yielded what is currently a highly credible theory of DAT.

Molecular Genetics of Huntington's Disease

The first dementing disease to yield up some of its secrets to molecular techniques was Huntington's disease. Through fragment-length polymorphisms, a disease-associated DNA segment was located on a far end of chromosome 4. Although this segment has not yet been isolated, its discovery had an important result that foreshadowed developments in other diseases. It is now possible to predict which persons among those at risk will develop the disease and which will not. This can be done from conception onward with an accuracy approaching 100 percent. The blessing is a mixed one, however, because there is as yet no way to treat the genetic defect, no way to prevent the development of this dread disease.

A multitude of ethical and human problems and opportunities have been uncovered by this combination of scientific breakthrough and lagging therapeutics. About half of those at risk decline testing because they don't want to know their fate. Providing psychological help and support to those who *do* wish to know and who then learn that they *will* develop the disease is a major preoccupation of the professions who deliver the results. In addition, the power to predict has created dilemmas that so far have not yielded to rational or ethical analysis. Does a person at risk have either a legal or a moral right to obtain blood from an unwilling family member if, as may well be the case, that blood is required for the risk to be determined? Should testing be done on underage persons? On those unborn? In the light of the fact that early Huntington's disease is associated with severe suicidal depression among other mental problems, what obligation to inform have professionals who know that a certain person destined to develop the disease has begun exhibiting eccentric or pathological behaviors that might be its first signs? These problems are just a sampler. The progression of biological science, like that of the physical sciences, seems certain to be marked by scientific breakthroughs that confer huge benefits but are intimately coupled with daunting human problems.

At present, genetic factors are the only known risk factor for primary dementias. However, genetics cannot provide a complete or sufficient explanation, and several other possible contributors are strong suspects. As described earlier, viral elements are an important contender, and we will explore their possible role in the next section.

Viruses

A virus is an extremely small organism, much smaller than a bacterium. It consists of genes and a coating of protein. When an infecting virus reaches the membrane of a cell, its genes enters the cell, leaving the virus's protein coat behind. The viral genes insert themselves into the genes of the host cell and then direct the cell to produce *viral* genes and proteins. The huge numbers of new viruses that are thus created, erupt from the host cell and go on in turn, to infect other cells. In many cases, the composition of the membrane of the target cells, which is determined by the host's genes, makes that membrane either more susceptible or less susceptible to penetration by viruses. In this way, and in other ways, genes affect the likelihood of viral infection.

Most viral infections—the common cold and measles, for example—develop and subside over a short time. Some serious infections of the brain (such as equine encephalitis) are due to viruses and also tend to have dramatic courses. But some viral infections are quite different. Instead of reproducing itself, the virus may lie dormant in the affected cell for years. Shingles, a common affliction due to the same virus as chicken pox, is an example of this process. Some viral infections may even be present at the birth of an organism but may not announce themselves for decades. Indeed, the biology of viruses and that of their hosts are most intricately intertwined. Viruses generally infect only one species; most human viruses do not infect other animals. Viruses cannot reproduce without their hosts, and they may permanently alter their hosts. Some of our genes, in fact, derived originally from infections. The invading genes were taken over by the regulatory machinery of cells belonging to our distant ancestors in the evolutionary chain and became established in our germ cell lines; now we use them to make products useful to ourselves. Much remains to be learned about the place of these parasitic agents in human ecology.

Some "slow" viruses, as those that lie dormant are termed, are known to affect the brain, and DAT has been regarded as a possible addition to the list. At present, the list includes:

○ Scrapie, a disease of sheep and goats

○ Kuru, a dementing illness limited to certain groups of natives of New Guinea

○ Creutzfeldt–Jakob disease, described briefly in
  Chapter 2

○ Gerstmann–Sträussler syndrome, a rare human
  disease

These infections appear to develop over considerable
periods of time—even over years—and to progress much more
slowly than most viral infections. They also lack fever and other
signs of acute illness, which distinguishes them from other
viral illnesses and makes their natural history difficult to
discover. They all produce a dementia which resembles the
dementia of the Alzheimer type.

The slow viruses also have a strong genetic component.
There are familial susceptibilities for all of them. Even kuru,
which seemed to be a purely environmental disease, apparently
has a genetic component. Transmission was thought to occur
through the eating of an infected human brain, a practice of
New Guinea tribes that is said to have been abandoned. However, kuru affected only about 50 percent of those who ate the
brain—a ratio highly suggestive of genetic suceptability.
Creutzfeldt–Jakob disease certainly "runs in families," and in
branches so far apart geographically that direct transmission
can be excluded. One form of Gerstmann–Sträussler syndrome
appears to be genetically transmitted, but a transmissible virus
produces a disease that is indistinguishable from the genetic
one. Moreover, all of the slow-virus infections listed above are
associated with a small protein, the prion, that appears in
infected cells and resembles amyloid in structure. The DNA
segment coding for the prion protein is located on human
chromosome 20. These relationships are far from settled. Puz-
zles abound.

One peculiarity of the slow viruses—scrapie serves as the
prototype—is that they have not been successfully grown in the
laboratory. Most viruses can be grown in eggs, but not scrapie.
Neither can the agent be seen or detected in any direct way.
Therefore, the only way to prove that viruses are in fact respon-

sible for these illnesses is actually to transmit them. To do this, brain tissue from an infected animal is fed to another animal (often a primate) or injected into its blood or brain. Years may have to pass before the disease appears. So far only Creutzfeldt–Jakob and kuru, among the diseases causing conditions that resemble DAT in humans, have been successfully transmitted in this way. However, the hypothesis is an attractive one to investigators, and several animals that have been exposed to tissue from other dementing illnesses, especially DAT, are still under observation.

It is possible that a viral contribution to some of the dementias described in Chapter 2 may eventually be proved. And meanwhile, because the virus itself cannot be shown to be present unless transmission occurs, the possibility is virtually impossible to *disprove*. Perhaps infection would develop in an exposed experimental animal if we waited longer, or perhaps there is some unknown reason why the exposures have not been effective. The fact that such possible reasons for failure always exist is a major logical hurdle; a useful scientific hypothesis must be testable, which means susceptible to being disproved. Nevertheless, attempts to demonstrate viral transmission continue. Investigators are sustained by the analogies to scrapie and Creutzfeldt–Jakob disease. Also, though the analogy to syphilis is seldom mentioned in scientific journals, there are striking resemblances between syphilitic infections of the brain and hypothetical slow-virus infections. Syphilis may lie dormant for many years before it produces brain disease that often includes features of dementia. Syphilis is caused not by a virus, but by a peculiar infectious agent, the spirochete, that was extremely difficult to detect through the first decades during which it was sought and that can still be difficult to detect. Finally, syphilis was once the single most frequent cause of brain disease, a position that DAT may occupy today. This is the more notable because a single genetic mechanism is most unlikely to produce disease in such a large proportion on the population. But infections do so regularly.

Neurotransmitters

Faulty communication among nerve cells has been implicated as contributing to dementing illness, and it provides the rationale for most modern attempts at treatment. This communication is accomplished through chemicals called neurotransmitters. It occurs at specific points (called synapses) on the surfaces of nerve cells (neurons). At a synapse, two nerve cells are very close to one another but do not touch; the tiny gap, is known as the synaptic cleft. A schematic diagram of a synapse appears in Figure 8.

The sending neuron contains neurotransmitters stored in small pockets called vesicles. When the sending neuron transmits, it discharges a neurotransmitter into the synaptic cleft, where that chemical affects special proteins, called receptors, in the surface membrane of the receiving neuron. When enough receptors are stimulated, the message is received. Most of the neurotransmitter is reabsorbed by the transmitting neuron, to be used again. The transmission of a nervous impulse is completed in milliseconds.

In the brain, the summation of these simple events becomes extremely complex. There are many different neurotransmitters, and every one of the billions of nerve cells in the brain is directly or indirectly connected to every other nerve cell. The surfaces of neurons are covered by synapses. A neuron receives messages from dozens—perhaps hundreds—of other neurons, probably via several neurotransmitters. It may send messages to a like number of other neurons. Neurotransmitters can stimulate the receiving neuron, making it more likely to respond, or they can inhibit it, making its response less likely to occur. Apparently, different neurotransmitters are often paired in systems in such a way that one neurotransmitter stimulates the response of a system as whole, and the other inhibits it.

Clearly, neurotransmission within the brain is extremely complex. But remember that our present understanding has developed over the past 10 to 15 years; progress has been extremely rapid. Already, some diseases are coming to be un-

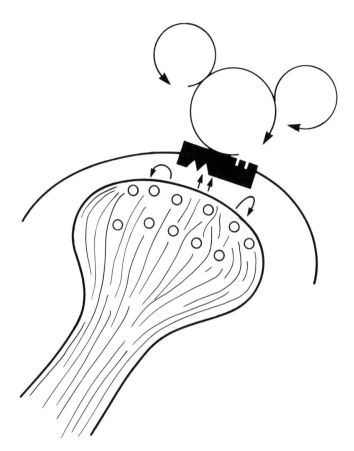

Figure 8 A synapse. The terminal of the nerve cell in the lower left of the figure stores neurotransmitters in vesicles represented by the circles within the cell. The neurotransmitter released fits precisely into a receptor molecule on the receiving cell. The unlocking of the receptor facilitates reactions within the receiving neuron. The neurotransmitter is then taken up by the transmitting neuron, to be used again later.

derstood in terms of a lack of sufficient neurotransmitter to stimulate the receiving membrane or a lack of receptors on that membrane. Parkinson's disease is marked by a lack of dopamine, a neurotransmitter at specific nerves. Huntington's disease may be associated with deficiencies in transmissions that require the neurotransmitter gamma amino butyric acid (GABA). Recently, it has become apparent that DAT features a decrease in the amount of another neurotransmitter, acetylcholine. In DAT, one group of neurons using acetylcholine to transmit nerve impulses may be selectively dying out.

Any fault in neurotransmission is likely to have a genetic basis, because genes instruct cells in how to make proteins. If the instructions are faulty, the protein might not do its job effectively. Some neurotransmitters are proteins; others are made by proteins. All neurotransmitters are positioned by proteins, all are discharged into the synaptic cleft by proteins, and most are reabsorbed to be stored by proteins. Receptors on the postsynaptic neuron are also proteins. The common thread is genetic relationships.

Aluminum

One of the consistent findings in autopsies of human victims of DAT is an excess of aluminum in their brains. The excess is extremely small; it can be detected only by the most sensitive instruments and after elaborate preparations. For example, special quartz beakers must be used preparing the tissue because enough aluminum to give spurious results would leach out of glass of even the highest quality. Questions have also been raised about the influence of aging on the concentration of aluminum. Its presence may be common in aged brains and not limited to those of persons afflicted with DAT. That possibility is being considered in current research projects.

Aluminum is abundant in nature, but its biological function, if any, is unknown. Like many other metals, it may participate in one or more chemical reactions as part of an enzyme, but because intense search has revealed no such function for aluminum, that seems most unlikely. Aluminum *can* induce in animals brain lesions that are similar to the neurofibrillary tangles seen in DAT. But the lesions are not identical and the difference is important. Many examples in the history of medicine tell us unequivocally that in tissue pathology, merely close is not close enough.

What the minute excess of aluminum in the brains of people who suffered from DAT may mean is not clear. It may become concentrated in the remaining brain tissue after the death and disappearance of nerve cells. (If this is so, aluminum would have nothing to do with the disease itself.) Or it may remain in tissue samples after destroying nerve cells. Those two possibilities suggest directly opposing explanations for the presence of excess aluminum in tissue. In fact, any biologist could devise a dozen other possible explanations and there would be no way to choose among them.

Because aluminum is so abundant in nature, we are constantly exposed to large amounts of it. The concentration of the metal in the tissues of experimental animals can be increased by feeding large amounts of it in the diet, but the origin of it in the brain in DAT is unlikely to be a dietary excess. If aluminum does contribute to the disease, some fault in the metabolic handling of the metal is much more likely to be responsible. Practically speaking, the aluminum hypothesis *requires* that such a fault exist because large numbers of people such as metal workers and persons taking certain medications have been exposed to massive amounts of aluminum in their environments without developing DAT. Conversely, DAT victims have not been found to have experienced extraordinary exposures to aluminum. Certainly there is no reason at all to avoid aluminum cookware or any other environmental source of aluminum.

Immune System

The immune system's function is to destroy or neutralize foreign material in the body. It destroys bacteria, viruses, foreign tissue of any kind, and even tissue that is normally present but has been transformed by injury or malignant change. The immune system is a foremost line of defense against disease. However, to do this job successfully, the im-

mune system must recognize normal body tissues and refrain
from destroying them. In other words, the system must be
regulated; it must be able to tell friend from foe. Some diseases
are the result of a failure of that very kind: the body attacks its
own tissue. The weapons used by the body's immune system
are proteins called antibodies. These are made by groups of
specialized lymphocytes, cells normally made in the bone mar-
row and released into the blood. Other lymphocytes regulate
the ones that make antibodies. There is some evidence that the
functioning of these regulating lymphocytes is impaired in
DAT.

One strong hint that immune system dysfunction may
be involved in DAT is the senile plaque itself. Amyloid is
present in tissue in so many immune system disturbances
that its presence in DAT at the very site of the injured tissue
strongly suggests an immune disorder. Some investigators
would substitute *proves* for *strongly suggests* in that statement, and would cite other supporting evidence as well. The
brain has some degree of ultimate control over the immune
system. Neurotransmitters almost certainly are involved in
immune responsiveness, so an impaired brain could be associated with an impaired immune system, and vice versa.
In addition, it has been claimed that actual antibodies
against brain tissue have been demonstrated in the circulating blood of persons with dementia. These antibodies increase in normal aging, but apparently the excess found in
dementia by some researchers is beyond what is normal.
Research in this area is difficult and the findings remain
equivocal, yet antibrain antibodies would provide a rational
explanation for progressive brain damage. They could
damage brain tissue by attaching to normal proteins, thus
interfering with the biological function of these proteins and
perhaps killing cells, including neurons.

The immune system, in all its complexity, is far from fully
understood. Many other possible disorders of its functions,
apart from the possible presence of antibrain antibodies, can
be postulated. It is a most logical place to look for dysfunction
in DAT and the other progressive dementias.

Hormonal Factors

A hormone is a chemical messenger that is secreted by one cell and has a biological effect on other, often very distant, cells. Neurotransmitters are hormones, though most represent special cases because they affect only cells immediately adjacent to cells producing them. The past decade has seen vast changes in our views of hormones and their place in biology. This is particularly true of hormones and the brain. Whole new classes of hormones secreted by brain tissue—the enkephalins—were discovered and are currently being investigated. In addition, other hormones have been found to influence learning and memory directly, and their possible contribution to dementia is being explored. Finally, very recently accumulated evidence suggests that other hormone systems are involved in the regulated growth and maintenance of neurons. Studies have so far yielded no results specifically relevant to DAT or other dementias, but these areas of inquiry are at the very frontier of research. Because changes in the life cycle such as menopause and aging, are associated with hormonal changes, the endocrine system is a promising place to look for causal factors in an age-related disease. One hormone, nerve growth factor (which we will discuss further in Chapter 6) is necessary for the maintenance of nerve cells in developing nervous tissue. As part of the programed development of the brain, nerve growth factor is withdrawn from populations of nerve cells, which thereupon die. This or analogous mechanisms could well contribute to dementia.

Medical Treatment and Management of Dementia

No medical treatment of the basic disease process has yet proved effective for any primary dementia. Even so, the atmosphere in medical research centers is one of expectancy: not that effective treatments will appear this year or next; but in ten years, quite possibly; in twenty years, likely. The reasons for such optimism will become apparent in this chapter. But in addition to supporting a hopeful outlook, the background knowledge supplied here will provide a basis for evaluating current attempts to treat the range of problems associated with dementing illness. Just avoiding the expense and heartbreak of resorting to treatments that are based on inadequate evidence or fraudulent claims could be a valuable benefit.

We emphasize that medicine is only one aspect of a treatment program. It is important for those dealing with dementing illness to develop a comprehensive plan as early as possible. This plan should be based on utterly realistic assessments of prognosis (what to expect from the illness); of the material resources that can be marshaled, including financial assets such as disability insurance, Social Security, and other pension plans; and, most of all, the availability and capabilities of human help. Of course, no plan can foresee all contingencies: Be sure that experience will force modifications, but the key is to begin. This chapter and the two that follow describe the basic ingredients of such a plan.

We begin by reviewing current attempts at direct treatment of dementia of the Alzheimer type (DAT) and Huntington's disease. Later in the chapter we outline practical management techniques that are useful when dealing with dementia.

Treatment of DAT

New research in DAT was given a great impetus by the demonstration that the activity of the enzyme known as choline acetyl transferase was greatly reduced in brain tissue from DAT victims. An enzyme is a protein that acts to catalyze (speed up) a specific chemical reaction. When an adequate amount of normally active enzyme is present, the chemical reaction that it facilitates proceeds at its biologically efficient rate. If enzyme activity is lacking, the rate is usually too slow or the reaction may not proceed at all. Choline acetyl transferase is vital to the chemical reaction that combines choline with an acetyl group to produce acetylcholine, a neurotransmitter. Remembering from Chapter 5 that communication between nerve cells depends on neurotransmitters, it stands to reason that lack of one would produce serious deficits in brain function. Acetylcholine is used by millions of nerve cells, so if communication involving them is impaired, mental activity is sure to be profoundly crippled.

Enzyme activity is usually measured by the amount of product (acetylcholine in this case) produced over a specified period of time. The amount of most products can be chemically measured, whereas it is generally not practical to measure the actual amount of enzyme. Therefore, there are several ways to explain reduced amounts of acetylcholine in brain tissue, including each of the following conditions:

1. Not enough choline acetyl transferase may be produced by brain cells even though the cells are present in normal numbers.

2. Enough choline acetyl transferase is produced but it is defective and thus not fully efficient.

3. Enough choline acetyl transferase is produced and it is fully effective, but there is not enough raw material (choline or acetyl or both) available for use in making the product.

4. Some cells that produce choline acetyl transferase have died for some unknown reason, and the remaining cells, though they produce enzyme with normal efficiency, cannot make up the loss.

5. Normal amounts of a normal enzyme are produced, but the enzyme is inactivated or destroyed before it can do its work.

These possibilities are being investigated in research laboratories. Meanwhile, the finding of decreased activity of choline acetyl transferase does suggest logical treatment trials which have been underway for the past decade. The first attempts, though crude, are important. They consisted mainly of giving large amounts of choline in the diet. While acetyl is present in ample amounts in the brain, choline must be supplied by other tissues or by diet. Thus if either component of acetylcholine is lacking (possibility 3 in the foregoing list), it probably will be choline. Moreover, if choline acetyl transferase is present in abnormally small amounts, or if its efficiency is somehow compromised (possibility 1 or 2), an extra supply of choline, coupled with the ample amounts of acetyl naturally present, could shift the normal equilibrium and force the production of additional acetylcholine. Many metabolic processes behave in such a way that the more raw material available, the more product is produced. If the product is lacking as a result of some disease, forcing the system to make more may lessen the signs and symptoms of the disease. That reasoning led to an effective treatment for Parkinson's disease (with L-dopa, a substance the brain uses to make the neurotransmitter dopamine), and it seemed worth trying in DAT.

Two methods of supplying added choline to the brain were tried. One was to give choline itself as a powder in capsules. The other was to give lecithin, a naturally occurring mixture of fatty substances rich in choline. Both methods delivered choline to the brain, but unknowns and drawbacks soon appeared. Optimal dosage was undetermined, though it was certainly large, and both choline and lecithin have characteristics that argue for finding a minimal effective dose. Choline in large doses produces side effects such as nausea, diarrhea, irritability, loss of appetite, and dry mouth. Lecithin produces much the same side effects, but the most important drawback of using lecithin is that it is a mixture of substances, only some of which are converted to choline by the body. In order to get enough choline, the patient had to take in about one-third of his or her total food calories as lecithin—a most unappetizing and expensive diet.

Of course, it would have been worth tolerating all these difficulties if only it could have been proved that getting more choline to the brain really helped. A grasp of how that question can be answered is crucial for anyone concerned with disease.

Principles of Treatment Evaluation

Determining whether or not a medical treatment works has proven endlessly troublesome, especially for chronic disease such as DAT. In DAT, diagnosis itself is problematic as we have noted. This has required meticulous screening of research subjects to reasonably ensure that they were indeed suffering from one of the primary progressive dementias. However, in the treatment trials so far conducted, specific diagnoses are rarely proved. The subjects may have had DAT or Pick's disease or any other dementing condition. Obviously, it is extremely difficult to assemble a treatment group and, sometimes much later, obtain autopsies to prove diagnoses. But not doing so risks the value of the study. The mixture of diseases being treated might well dilute even a significant positive response of an experimental treatment, making it undetectable.

Diagnosis is far from the only problem. Another is how improvement due to an experimental treatment should be measured. At present in dementia research, this is done mainly by administering psychological tests before and after treatment. Improvement in the test scores, or at least an absence of the worsening scores expected over time in primary dementia constitutes positive outcome. In practice, doing this research is much more difficult than it seems. The easiest tests are difficult enough so that persons with even a moderate dementia cannot score high enough to be tested. And, of course, there is a certain amount of error inherent in the test scores; that is, subjects might obtain any score within a limited range just by chance. Furthermore, practice helps, so the second administration of a test after a period of treatment might produce a misleadingly high score. Test scores may also be influenced by a large number of factors not related to the disease or its treatment, including time of day, distractions in the environment, the personality of the examiner, minor physical discomfort, and mood. Finally, there is the insidious placebo effect. Performance can be boosted just by the subject's awareness of having been given an experimental drug that subjects, examiners, medical personnel, and all others concerned fervently hope will prove effective.

Such cautionary notes might seem unnecessarily picky, but medical research has been led astray many times by each of the factors mentioned above and by many others like them. This has led to the adoption of standard research designs for treatment trials. The basic element in these designs is the placebo control. Instead of the experimental drug, another substance, a placebo, is administered to members of a control group. The placebo may be either an inactive drug (such as a sugar), or one that is known to be ineffective against the disease being treated but has definite physical effects, so that subjects will know they are taking something active. In all other respects, the control group and the experimental group are treated exactly alike. Often new drugs are tested against standard treatments; if so the design usually includes three phases: old drug, new drug, placebo. Of course, there is no standard treatment, or "old drug" available for comparison in the dementing illnesses. This is an important deficit. Even a marginally effective treatment would provide a most helpful comparison, a baseline level of efficacy that new treatments would have to surpass.

Other design features are standard in pharmacology. Placebo capsules or tablets must look exactly like those containing the active drug. All concerned should be "blind;" that is, no patient, doctor, nurse, or family member, nor anyone else connected with the treatment team should know whether a placebo or the experimental drug is being given to any subject. One or two people associated with the project but not involved with the treatment hold that information in coded form until the study is complete and analysis of the results begins. As approaches to a disease are refined, it may become clear that stronger designs with additional safeguards are required. One that is commonly used is the crossover. A patient-subject is given the drug or placebo for a set period of time and then, for a like period, is given the drug if placebo was given before and vice versa. All assignments to treatment and placebo groups are made randomly so that any subject is equally likely to be given placebo as the experimental treatment.

Lay persons should be aware of these principles of research design. The temptation to try something—anything—that might just possibly help combat a disease such as DAT is extremely strong, and unproven remedies abound. These are nearly always expensive, and some are dangerous. Use common sense and inquire whether the principles of research design described above were applied in testing any treatment recommended. It will never be possible to achieve perfect rationality when trying to cope with diseases that have catastrophic consequences, and any of us might lean further than is rational in the direction of hope. But we just must try our best not to lean so far that we lose our balance and fall. That helps no one.

Another reason why family members should be well informed about the methods employed in drug trials is that anyone who has a dementing illness is likely to be asked to participate in one. Because dementia itself lessens one's competency to decide questions such as whether or not to participate in a drug trial, relatives are often asked to participate in the decision. It is the responsibility of the research team to explain exactly what questions the research project seeks to answer and how those answers are to be obtained. There are a few guidelines to help the lay person gauge the worth of a project. Nearly all projects supported by private foundations or government funds are reviewed by independent scientists (in a process known as peer review) and also by an independent and broadly representative Human Subjects Committee charged with ensuring that the project meets ethical standards and that any risk to participants is warranted by advances in understanding that the research might yield. It is quite proper to inquire about the funding of a project and to ask whether or not a Human Subjects Committee has reviewed it. A project that has passed those reviews is probably scientifically worthwhile and safe to participants. However, many worthwhile projects are not supported by grants, and while most will have been reviewed by a Human Subjects Committee, in the end, it may be necessary to apply the standards above leavened by good common sense.

If a project seems worthwhile scientifically and reasonably safe, by all means encourage participation in it. There is a surprising shortage of willing subjects who qualify for promising studies, especially in placebo-controlled trials of treatment. Remember, no one can know into which group a subject will be placed, and some subjects will receive only placebos. This is often hard to accept. If there is the slightest chance that a treatment may be successful, no one wants to be assigned to prove it by getting worse taking a placebo. Yet there is no other way if anyone at all is to benefit. Too, modern studies nearly always provide active treatment for all subjects at some time. That is, every subject who is initially given a placebo eventually gets the experimental drug. And, of course, whenever a treatment is proven effective, all participants will be given the active drug.

Choline and Lecithin

Let us now look at how research into choline and lecithin treatments fared in light of the standards explained above. Several completed studies have been placebo-controlled; none have included crossovers. By and large, no benefits were demonstrated. However, a few subjects did seem to improve, if only slightly. Singling out a few subjects who seemed to improve would be unacceptable in trials of other drugs in other diseases. Nevertheless, such results are regarded as a wisp of hope in DAT research because the theoretical basis of the treatment is sound and because without treatment the disease worsens. Thus any improvement at all, even in a small proportion of subjects, suggests that just maybe the drug being given should not be discarded. Perhaps the best evaluation of the effectiveness of choline and lecithin treatments have not been proved to fail. It is not that these treatments are likely to succeed, but simply that the theory underlying them may have merit and that improved drugs of the same class should be sought.

Today, active trials are underway involving 15 different drugs that aim to increase the level of acetylcholine in the brain. This new generation of drugs was suggested by trials of choline and lecithin and by the known pharmacology of the venerable drug, physostigmine. The aim in giving these drugs is preventing the destruction of acetylcholine. It currently seems to be along that front that DAT promises to be most vulnerable.

Physostigmine

This drug, the prototype of the group, prevents the destruction of acetylcholine. If acetylcholine is needed for memory formation, then physostigmine might improve memory, and in fact it does just that, though to a marginal extent, in normal young persons. It has been tried in DAT, but the results have so far been disappointing. Unfortunately, physostigmine is a most difficult drug to study. It is so toxic that it can be given only in minute doses and only by injection. A single injection is active in the brain for only a short time—probably just seconds. For all these reasons, current pharmacological research on DAT is aimed at developing a drug that acts like physostigmine but can be taken by mouth, has a longer duration of action, and is acceptably safe. Remember: Physostigmine's effect on memory is slight and short-lived, while its other actions can quickly produce death. Do not experiment with this drug.

THA (Tetrahydroaminoacridine)

Testing is nearly completed on one drug with physostigmine-like action, and the preliminary results are promising. The drug is tetrahydroaminoacridine, popularly known by the initials THA. It is important to distinguish between treatments that improve the immediate signs and symptoms of DAT and those that prevent long-term progression of the disease. THA is being tested only for its effectiveness in improving short-term memory. The improvement so far associated with the drug is slight, but it has apparently been proved, and safety has been reasonably ensured. The drug will soon be available. Meanwhile, other preparations with similar properties are being tested. The evolution of these new products should improve the treatments available.

The testing of THA has provided valuable lessons and experience. The study was a massive and complicated one: The work was done in several research centers across the United States. It was organized and funded by a cooperative effort among two U.S. agencies (the Food and Drug Administration and the National Institute on Aging), a volunteer advocacy group (the Alzheimer's Disease Association), and a drug company (Warner-Lambert). This coordinated effort permitted rapid and effective testing of a promising drug.

A preparation that mimics the action of physostigmine, but is chemically only related to THA distantly, has been available for several years. This is aercholine. Although it is relatively free of toxicity, other side effects of aercholine discourage its use for ongoing treatment. It must be administered by injection, and it induces nausea and vomiting in most people. Like physostigmine, aercholine is a starting point for the development of new drugs, some of which are being tested.

Different premises underlie research into other drugs. The drug actions involved and the rationale for their use in treating DAT is unclear. They range from aminopyridines (drugs that block potassium channels in cells) through nootropics (which purport to enhance cellular metabolism) to GABA agonists (preparations that in some manner increase or mimic the effects of the neurotransmitter gamma aminobutyric acid). There are no compelling reasons to think that any of these preparations will prove effective. Current research is based on hints at best, the strongest probably supporting the nootropics, known as piracetam and oxiracetam.

Those are the treatments currently being investigated and discussed for DAT. Several other approaches have been made to treating the dementias in general and are not targeted specifically at DAT. All of these treatments have either practical or theoretical applications, and some have both.

Hydergine

This preparation is actually a mixture of drugs related to ergot. It is widely used in geriatric populations, especially in Europe. Evaluation of its effectiveness is difficult because Hydergine probably has an elevating effect, though a slight one, on mood. It may possibly have a very marginal effect on mental functioning, but current thinking holds that this effect, if it exists, is secondary to the effect on mood. (When mood brightens even a little, some positive effects on mental function can be expected.) That interpretation is consistent with the available evidence.

Neuropeptides

A group of proteins known as neuropeptides are secreted by brain tissues and change the operating characteristics of other cells at distant locations. These peptides (a peptide is a short segment of a protein) act in every way as hormones act. For example, one such peptide appears to be secreted by one group of neurons in response to pain. It then acts on another group of neurons to diminish the intensity of the organism's experience of pain. This neat and efficient method evolved by nature enables an injured organism to continue functioning in an emergency. Why, then, shouldn't other peptides modify the operating characteristics of other groups of neurons? Mood is one obvious possibility. Especially intriguing are peptides that appear to exert on neurons a tonic effect that may be essential to the continuing health of nervous tissue. Such essential maintenance functions have been found generally in tissues; for example, weight bearing is required for maintenance of bone calcification. Though no such functions have so far been discovered for the brain, their existence can hardly be doubted.

Peptide systems on which experimental work is proceeding have been found to affect the maintenance of nerve cells. An example is nerve growth factor, a peptide without which nerve cells die. Normal development of the embryonic and infantile brain requires that some nerve cells die. Because development is an ongoing process throughout life, including involutional changes that accompany aging, aberrations in peptide mechanisms such as nerve growth factor offer promising directions in which to search for causes.

Evidence links other peptides directly to memory and learning. ACTH 4–10, for example, seems to enhance mental performance, including memory. It is actually a short segment that appears in each of two much longer protein hormones: vasopressin and adrenocorticotropic hormone (hence ACTH). This situation appears to be common in biology. During the course of evolution, the genes coding for ancestral proteins were duplicated several times by accident. This duplication provided extra genes that were not needed for ongoing life processes and were thus available for change through mutation. By taking advantage of opportunity, as animals which survive the course of evolution generally do, new hormones apparently were fashioned using the extra genes.

The study of peptides is just beginning. There appear to be dozens of them and at least as many suggested functions. So far, only ACTH4–10 has been tested in human populations. Although it does enhance mental efficiency in normals, it does not appear to benefit suffers of primary dementia. Years of laboratory research will be needed before these hormone systems are well understood. But the reward may be very great indeed.

That exhausts the list of treatments and possible treatments for DAT that are currently of scientific interest. Even if we knew them all, listing all the treatments that have been advocated or actually tried and found useless would add little light. Some that have enjoyed public acclaim in the past are procaine by injection, metrazol, low-cholesterol or low-fat diets, papaverine, and anticoagulants (which prevent blood clots from forming). Two other, more recent treatments should be mentioned: hyperbaric oxygen and massive doses of vitamins. Oxygen at high pressure was briefly claimed to have dramatic effects in restoring brain function. However, this claim has been decisively discredited. Vitamins have been advocated by enthusiastic partisans for virtually all brain diseases, including progressive dementia. There is a definite place for vitamin therapy in secondary dementias, some of which are associated with nutritional deficiencies. Physicians are generally aware of this possibility and order tests to establish whether vitamin deficiencies exist. If there is no such deficiency, administering more vitamins is quite useless.

Quackery

Desperate people grasp at straws, and dementing illness invites desperation. There have always been those who exploit the despair engendered by illness. Some genuinely believe in their remedies with conviction that borders on fanaticism. Others are frankly frauds. Until effective treatments are found for DAT and like illnesses, quackery will flourish.

Two widely advertised treatments for DAT will serve as examples of quackery. One, known as corticosuppression treatment is based on the assumption that adrenocorticotropic hormone is produced in excess in DAT. The advertisements we have seen are quite disarming. They make it clear that there is no evidence whatsoever supporting this theory of the cause of DAT or suggesting that the proposed treatment might do any good. Nevertheless, the ads recommend the treatment. Lawyers have done a skillful job of protecting their exploitive clients from charges of making unfounded claims while implying, simply by advocating the treatment, that it is worthwhile. We heartily endorse the disclaimers. Neither the theory of DAT advanced nor the proposed treatment is supported by the slightest bit of evidence.

The same evaluation is warranted for chelation therapy. This theory is based on the presence of aluminum in brain tissue (see Chapter 5). Chelators are chemical compounds that attach to metals and remove them from tissues. Clearly, there is a defensible rationale for trying chelation in the treatment of DAT, and scientifically credible trials are underway. However, far in advance of whatever results will emerge, quacks have been promoting chelation therapy. In this case, the treatment as administered not only has the usual trappings of quackery, ineffectiveness and great expense, but is also dangerous. Chelators don't discriminate among metals, and treatment results in the loss of essential ones, especially calcium and magnesium. Expert medical attention is required, and even then, safe treatment requires delicate management.

Treatment of Huntington's Disease

Huntington's disease is the only other progressive dementia for which a rationale for treatment has been developed. In brain tissue from victims of the disease, there is a deficiency of the neurotransmitter gamma aminobutyric acid (GABA). And the enzyme that makes GABA, glutamic acid decarboxylase, is also present in low concentration. Accordingly, certain drugs have been given reasonably sophisticated trials. Musciniol, which might directly substitute for GABA, was found to be ineffective. So was Depakine, which slows the normal breakdown of GABA.

While no direct treatment of the dementing process has yet proven effective in Huntington's disease, the severity of the movement disorder, which itself is quite disabling, can be helped quite a lot. The drugs that best accomplish this are phenothiazines, or major tranquilizers. These drugs act by blocking the receptors for the neurotransmitter dopamine. It is thought that nerve cells activated by dopamine and GABA, respectively, have opposite effects. Thus, the theory goes, a deficiency of GABA leaves dopamine to act unopposed; the normal balance is upset and symptoms result. This explanation will probably turn out to be much too simple. But as a hypothesis, it is enormously more sophisticated than anything that could have been suggested a few short years ago.

Management: General Principles

Effective and humane management of the environment and needs of the person suffering from dementing illness requires great practical ingenuity and great compassion. No guidelines can cover the specific circumstances encountered with each victim. Even so, certain general principles derived from observation of and interaction with many families coping with dementia, should be helpful. We offer them here.

Interactions with a person who has a progressive dementia must be based on constant awareness of the mental capacity remaining. Early in the course (say 3 to 4 years after onset), affected persons are generally aware of their memory deficit, but most tend strongly to minimize or deny it. Direct confrontation is usually not helpful in such instances Patience is needed, but most affected persons eventually begin to participate in management of the disease. Even so, reactions to dementia differ greatly from person to person, and we know of no general rules for obtaining the patient's cooperation. Use your knowledge of the ill person's personality.

Affected persons may not be the only ones who have trouble recognizing that an illness is present. Frustrating and agonizing months may pass before those in daily contact with a person in the early stages of a progressive dementia grasp what is happening and are ready to begin adapting to it. Spouses in particular often seem unable or unwilling to come to grips with the new realities. To others who are directly though not so immediately concerned—grown children for example—the increasing mental impairment often seems more obvious. Disagreements at this stage can be quite painful.

Let us suppose it is the husband who is developing progressive dementia. His wife either does not seem to comprehend the change or offers inadequate explanations of it: "After all, we are all getting older." "He has just had so much on his mind." The couple's children, however, who are usually in their thirties and forties, realize that something is wrong. What should they do?

A Visit to the Doctor

First, get medical help as soon as possible. See that a general examination is scheduled and give the physician the facts that underlie your suspicions. Sometimes physicians can act very effectively as objective assessors of the situation the family faces. Meanwhile, resist any temptation to confront the wife directly: "Look, Mom, he bought salt for the water softener three times last week." Rather, bring up such an example from time to time to illustrate the developing impairment, but don't repeat it often, and most of all don't insist that the wife acknowledge its import.

To develop insights helpful in dealing with the wife in such situations, try to think of her problem as separated into two broad components. By far the more difficult aspect of the problem for any spouse of an individual who has a dementing illness is witnessing the progressive disintegration of the personality of the person with whom he or she has shared much of life. Recognizing that a loved one is no longer the person he or she was, and never again will be, is very painful for most spouses. Arriving at that acceptance takes time and cannot be rushed by confrontation. The other component of the problem the spouse faces is the need to recognize and adapt to the loss of the ill husband or wife as a full partner in the management of the household. This means the wife we are discussing will have to assume more and more of her husband's duties or see that responsibility for them is effectively delegated. This is the easier part for most families, and the need for it arises earlier in the disease. Tackle it first.

Of course, a husband faces similar problems when his wife suffers from dementia. However, one major difference between their situations affects the generation now at risk (though perhaps not the next one). Today, the husband whose wife has a dementing illness is more often still working and must juggle the care of his wife with the demands of his job. In practice, few men can manage this. Early retirement is often the most humane choice and also (because home care is so very expensive) the best financial arrangement.

No matter whether a woman or a man is affected, getting the ill person to give up specific tasks is relatively easy. When we are confronted with situations that we cannot grasp, we become anxious. The signs of anxiety include increasing agitation—fidgeting, purposeless movements, expressed desire to leave the situation, and (most of all) decreasing mental competence. Be alert for such signs and do not discount them. Anxiety itself can start a vicious circle: It interferes with effective functioning, which leads to more anxiety, which further impairs functioning, and so on. Because anxiety is an extremely aversive emotion that we go to great lengths to avoid, the dementing person is powerfully motivated to escape anxiety. This simple fact of human experience is a great help to those who need to get a victim of dementia to relinquish certain responsibilities. Mental tasks beyond the person's capacity produce anxiety. The anxiety is usually attached to specific tasks, however, so avoid generalizing deficits. Be specific and concrete. Say to the wife described above, "He can't balance the checkbook, so you will have to start doing that." Avoid such generalizations as: "You will have to start managing the money."

Welcome relief from anxiety generally makes it reasonably easy to get the dementing person to yield control to others of tasks such as balancing the checkbook. It also helps deciding when to retire from work because dementing persons are nearly always aware of their failure to achieve their previous standards, and that provokes anxiety. Unless the work is intrinsically dangerous—mixing chemicals or flying, for example—it is usually safe to rely on increasing anxiety to signal the proper time to withdraw from it.

One exception to this general rule that often proves especially troublesome is driving. People tend *not* to become anxious about their ability to drive safely and continue far too long. Forceful action may be required of relatives. Physicians can help, because in many states they can file a simple report that will result in suspension of the driving license. This technically solves the problem, but practical enforcement of a driving ban sometimes remains the responsibility of family members. If necessary, hide the keys. Never ever leave them in the ignition.

No Need for Stimulation

In the earlier stages of a dementing process, which in many ways are the most difficult ones, it may seem natural to apply a bit of traditional wisdom that we regard as misguided. The underlying idea is that the brain should be exercised just as muscles are: "Keep the brain active in order to keep it from atrophying. Use it or lose it." This is wrong. The brain is not like muscle. It will stay active so long as it is healthy. By all means, try to keep ill persons interested in the world around them as long as possible. However, being too zealous about this can overburden a deteriorating brain with consequent increasing anxiety and decreasing efficiency. Only if a depressed mood is a part of the overall problem is there some reason, though even then not a very good one, to artificially stimulate interest and activity. Again, the ill person is probably the best available guide. If he or she consistently seeks to withdraw from stimulation, don't try to prevent it.

Progressive dementia is accompanied by progressive withdrawal from social activities. The basic ideas outlined above apply with special force here. Social occasions can be difficult. Keep the numbers of new faces and new names to a minimum. Social conversations tend to focus on current events, and short-term memory is the dementing person's greatest weakness. Help by judiciously supplying answers and the steering conversation toward safer topics; reminisce unabashedly. Again, and most of all, be aware of developing anxiety. Virtually any sign of discomfort is a signal that capacity is at or fast approaching overload.

The Value of Familiar Routines

Eventually dementia makes learning new material an ordeal not worth its cost, and the ill person seeks to avoid such demands. By all means, allow this withdrawal. However, brief social events limited to a few familiar faces, and without distractions such as unfamiliar surroundings or noise from active children, are likely to be pleasurable to all concerned. Guard against overestimating the affected person's mental capacity; doing so is much more common than underestimating what she or he can tolerate and enjoy.

In daily life, try to maintain a routine that features well established landmarks such as regular meals. Make life predictable. Avoid breaks in routine whenever possible, and be especially mindful of the total dose of disruption over time. If some disturbance of routine is necessary, minimize its intensity. Do not concentrate changes. Instead, extend any necessary changes over as long a period of time as possible. In general, be matter-of-fact in conversation. Avoid ambiguity and, in particular, do not present unnecessary choices or decisions. Say, "Now we must go to the store," not "Would you like to come to the store with me?" Always be concrete. Say, "Alan is coming to visit after lunch," not "We are going to have company today." Give positive direction. Say, "Now it is time to take a shower," not "Shall we eat now or would you rather take a shower first?"

Try to maintain the victim of dementia in familiar surroundings—the more familiar the better. This includes keeping the home environment as constant as possible. Don't rearrange all of the furniture in a room. Don't even let newspapers or other litter accumulate. Dramatic change, such as moving to a new residence, can bring on disastrous decompensation. When one has lived in the same place for many years, there is a limited amount of new information to be assimilated each day. But in new surroundings, one has to learn where every light switch is located and the simplest geography of the rooms. Probably we have all had the experience of suddenly—perhaps on awakening in the middle of the night—of being unaware of where we are, and we have found the experience intensely anxiety provoking for a moment or two. Normally, we recover quickly and no harm is done. But for the sufferer from dementia who can't retain information, there may be no such quick recovery because he or she can't retain enough information to quickly reorient. Increasing anxiety, paired with the resulting decreased ability to reason, launches a vicious circle that can lead to a confusional psychosis. Recovery from such an episode occurs within a few days, but it is an experience to be avoided. If a move is absolutely essential, schedule it as early in the illness as possible to take advantage of whatever intellectual reserves remain, or delay the move as long as possible to minimize awareness of the change in surroundings. Bringing along as many familiar things as possible helps. Keep old familiar furniture and furnishings.

Avoidance of Fatigue and Ambiguity

Fatigue is poorly tolerated by victims of dementia, but it can generally be avoided. Schedule trying activities, such as visits to doctors, to occur after a period of sleep. Encourage frequent rests. Even an hour of activity may be excessive in some cases, and a period of rest may be remarkably restorative. Above all, do not schedule several hours of unbroken activity.

In addition to planning ahead to avoid hazards, there are positive things to do. Get good at "reorienting" the one you are caring for. Do this by remaining aware at all times of the main disability in order to compensate for it with your own memory. Consider an occasion when the grandchildren are visiting. Suppose they are playing in the next room, and suddenly you hear a noise there. Your healthy brain remembers instantly that the children are there and concludes: "Oh, the children are in the next room; they explain the noise. It does not sound dangerous. They're just playing." But for the brain that cannot remember what is going on in the next room, such sudden noises are unexplained, and cause alarm and anxiety. Being aware of this, upon hearing the noise you simply remark softly, "That is the children playing in the next room. They are OK."

In the next section, we offer some suggestions for dealing with certain more specific problems that arise in the management of dementia.

Management: Some Specifics

There is much that families who prepare themselves can do to increase the comfort and safety of the dementia patient and to make the household run smoothly. Drugs may sometimes be an appropriate treatment when such symptoms as anxiety and wandering at night become a problem. But establishing effective practices in the management of such activities as toileting are also important.

Drug Treatments for Symptoms

Management of dementia is usually made much easier by the judicious use of medications to control symptoms. However, the problems encountered are not simple. The elderly, especially those affected with dementing illness, are often extremely sensitive to drugs. Their systems do not dispose of drugs as quickly as younger persons on whom standard dosages are based, so it is possible for successive doses to accumulate in older persons and produce unexpected toxicity. Side effects are also more likely to develop in older persons, and they tend to be unusually severe. Unfortunately, most of the drugs used to minimize the symptoms of dementia are difficult to manage. Moreover, elderly people differ widely in their response to drugs, much more widely in fact than younger people. This means that both choosing drugs and finding the right dose become effectively empirical: that is, what is right depends more on outcome than on pharmacologic theory. Prudent medical practice emphasizes one overriding generalization in prescribing drugs and setting the dosage for elderly patients: "Start low and go slow."

At some point, usually early in the course of dementing illness, belligerence or anxiety may become troublesome enough to require treatment with drugs. If so, prescription drugs are needed, and the neuroleptic drugs (tranquilizers) are quite efficient in reducing problem behavior. Usually only very small doses are needed—on the order of 10 to 25 milligrams of chlorpromazine (Thorazine), or an equivalent dosage of another drug in the same class (a phenothiazine, or major tranquilizer). However, even small doses often produce side effects in the elderly. Ask your doctor about side effects, especially extrapyramidal or Parkinsonian effects, and what you should do about them. Extrapyramidal side effects are mainly muscular rigidity, which may produce both stiffness and bizarre posturing, and tremor that often resembles that of Parkinson's disease. In our experience, other drugs that are effective in alleviating agitation or anxiety, such as diazepam (Valium), can be most useful, even though they may produce mild intoxication and interfere with memory formation. These drugs may also produce addiction, but overall, they do not deserve their bad reputation in this regard. Most often, it is necessary to experiment with several drugs and dosages in order to arrive at optimal benefit. Once this happy state is reached, think in terms of reducing the dosage in small steps while being prepared to increase again if needed. As the disease progresses, lower doses will ordinarily suffice.

Nocturnal wandering, common in dementia, can prove very troublesome, especially because others in the home must sleep. Give whatever sedation is needed. Most often, the neuroleptic drugs (tranquilizers) are prescribed for sleep, and they are effective and safe. However, their action is long-lasting, so the effects of an evening dose may persist through the next day. That may be either a wanted or an unwanted effect. Several benzodiazepine drugs (members of the same class as Valium) have short durations of action and are often the better choice. Encourage your doctor to experiment judiciously; then observe the results and be guided accordingly. Finally, if evening sedation is used, avoiding fluid intake for the three to four hours before bedtime may be a useful precaution against bedwetting or attempts to get to the bathroom while impaired by sedation.

Cramps and Seizures

Earlier we mentioned muscle cramps and generalized seizures as fairly common complications in the later stages of dementing illness. Unfortunately, the conventional treatments for these conditions are usually unsatisfactory. We do advise avoiding fatigue for both conditions; cramps in particular seem to be associated with fatigue. We also advise trying propranolol (Inderal) for cramps or for tremors which may develop as the illness progresses.

Bowel and Bladder Hygiene

Another issue that often arises is bowel and bladder hygiene. Constipation is a very common problem for the elderly. In dementia, it may become especially troublesome because of inattention or medication. The first remedy is to ensure that fluid intake is adequate—a simple, important step, that is too often neglected. Second, maintain regular bowel habits. The ill person should sit on the toilet at the same time each day, usually in the morning just after a meal. If constipation persists, daily administration of a drug such as Colase often solves the problem. If not, it is best to get medical help.

Actual loss of control of bowel and bladder can be anticipated in dementia. Incontinence is the single development that most often leads to placement in a nursing home. For that reason, and for the greater comfort of both patient and family, continence should be preserved as long as possible. Urinary control can also be helped by routine toileting. The urinary stream can often be started by exerting gentle pressure over the urinary bladder (just above the pubic bone) or by gently stroking the inner surface of the thigh. Women, especially those who have had a catheter in place for some reason, sometimes lose bladder control earlier than is usually observed to be associated with the degree of dementia present. A menstrual pad may prove helpful in such cases.

Sex

As dementing illness progresses, interest in sex usually diminishes. Some persons may become hypersexual, and though this is rare, it may appear or reappear at different times during the illness. Most often the object of the attention is the spouse, but sometimes other persons in the home or neighborhood may be approached. This may require close attention, not so much because the behavior is likely to be dangerous, but because it may well be perceived as dangerous and cannot be ignored. If sexual behavior threatens to be troublesome, consult a physician. Control is usually quite easy to attain.

In the early stages of the illness, some people may become preoccupied with sexual concerns and use inappropriate language, even if this behavior is entirely alien to the personality exhibited before the illness began. Sometimes sexual paranoia may appear. A spouse may be accused of having an affair, and mistrust may extend to the most casual social conversation. Yet within a short time, the same person can become so remorseful as to cry because of the accusations made. Such mistaken ideas are rarely held for any length of time and are hardly ever of dangerous intensity. Ignore such incidents and try to divert the affected person's interest to other things. Generally no harm at all will be done.

Vision and Hearing

You want to give the victim of dementia every possible break, so even apparently small points should not be overlooked. Ensure adequate input to the senses. Light can be extremely important. Older persons lose visual acuity, making the surroundings appear dim. A normal brain can largely compensate for this loss by supplying from memory any details of the environment that are imperfectly perceived. An impaired brain cannot do this so well, and the familiar vicious circle may be set into play: Uncertainty leads to anxiety, which leads to increased uncertainty, which in turn leads to panic. Unusually intense lighting kept on all night at strategic locations may help prevent this; hallways, stairs, and bathrooms are likely candidates in most homes. Usually it pays to buy and install fluorescent fixtures. Fluorescent lights are sufficiently intense, are relatively free of distortion, and can be kept on for hours at little cost. Unlike incandescent lights, fluorescent lights use little current when operating. Power is drawn when they are first turned on. But when they are left on, the fluorescent bulbs last a very long time and power use is minimal.

Sound is also important. It often helps to have a radio tuned to a station that plays old familiar tunes. This is an old remedy, well known to hospitals and nursing staffs. It is worth trying. However, if hearing is impaired, a hearing aid is not often useful in dementia. Apparently, making the adjustment to an aid, which is often difficult even for normal elderly persons, is nearly impossible in dementia. Remember too, that ambiguous stimuli such as distracting noises of uncertain origin are to be strictly avoided.

Safety

We have found that most dementing persons are not at major risk from household hazards. Some are, however, and it is important to couple the degree of disability present at a given time with sensible preventive measures needed to safeguard the ill person's environment. Here are a few hints. Application of common sense about fire and electricity is usually sufficient. If you are uneasy, mounting a smoke alarm in every room offers effective and cheap reassurance. Consider removing control dials and levers from stoves. Be sure that you can unlock all interior doors from both sides, and have one or more rooms, as well as dangerous areas such as the garage or basement, equipped with locks that can be opened only with keys that you keep. Hide a house key outdoors so that you can't be locked out, and never never never leave automobile keys in the ignition lock. Lock medicines and alcohol away.

Wandering can be a problem. Sew name-and-address labels into clothing. Conventional measures used in many hospitals to prevent wandering, such as removing shoes and keeping the victim dressed in pajamas, do not help at home. Alarms on critical doors can be helpful. Many ill persons obey without question signs such as "STOP." Try placing a few. A MEDALERT bracelet giving name, address, telephone number, and bearing the inscription "memory loss" is a good idea.

Most of all, human help is needed. Neighbors will usually help control wandering. However, the dementing person will eventually require supervision for each one of the twenty-four hours in each day. He or she will have to be protected and will have to be toileted, dressed, and fed. Some arrangements will have to be made to relieve the primary caregiver—usually the spouse. Not much can be done to lessen the problem. Spouses vary greatly in their dedication and resolve, but many tend to "go it alone" far too long. The rest of the family may have to impose the needed help. Act soon rather than later. Finally, the victim of a dementing illness will require care in a medical facility, usually a nursing home. The next two chapters will take up that and related subjects.

CHAPTER 7

Hospitals, Nursing Homes, and Care Alternatives

We noted earlier that dementia often first appears when the routine of everday living is changed. For example, a family vacation in unfamiliar surroundings may elicit early symptoms of dementing illness. Change in surroundings and constant movement can be confusing for all of us; for the person with dementia, the confusion can be overwhelming.

Because change in environment is a major source of stress for persons with dementia, their condition may worsen when they enter a hospital or other care facility. Besides the change in physical environment, they must contend with changes in personnel, and visits to unfamiliar locations to undergo tests. The patient may become confused, disoriented, and lost. And relatives may be upset to find their loved one uncooperative or verbally abusive, wandering the halls, refusing to eat, shouting, and sometimes behaving violently. Confused persons may harm themselves—for example, by pulling out intravenous tubes. Visits may be stressful. Faced with this, family members may conclude that they themselves can provide better care and that their relative would be better off at home. In a way they are right.

Hospitalization of an elderly person for any reason can cause a decline in mental status. A heart attack, major surgery, and a broken hip are examples of catastrophic medical or surgical events that may be associated with abrupt deterioration of mental functioning. The illness or injury, and the following hospitalization, acts as a major environmental stressor. As healing progresses, and especially when it becomes possible to return home, mental status generally improves. But recovery may take a long time and it may not be complete: "She was never the same after the accident." In such cases, the reserve capacity of the brain may have been exceeded. It is also possible, of course, that an incipient deficit in mental functioning contributed to the illness or injury that led to hospitalization.

No matter how stressful, hospitals and nursing homes are almost certain to be needed during a dementing illness, so becoming acquainted with the services they offer is an important aspect of planning. Caring for persons with a dementing illness is a 24-hour, 7-day-a-week job. Taking care of the victim at home can become overwhelming. Alternatives should be investigated *before* the caregiver's burden becomes intolerable, and the caregiver should not decide on an alternative alone; the family should participate. A doctor's recommendation supporting the primary caregiver's need for relief, is important if there are relatives who may not understand how difficult the situation has become. To some, it may seem that the dementia is not "bad enough" to warrant outside care, and this difference of opinion can lead to accusations and feelings of guilt. In general, the more the whole family shares the responsibility for such major decisions, the better the primary caregiver and the patient are served. Emotional support from the entire family can significantly ease transitions demanded by the progression of the disease.

It is true that major changes permanently affect many people with dementia. Yet many other victims of dementing illness adjust satisfactorily, and although their condition may slowly worsen, they are reasonably happy in the new environment. Time helps.

The alternatives to patient care at home provided by a family member include hospitalization of the patient, various kinds of short-term relief for the primary caregiver (known as respite care), and long-term care. For the reasons outlined below, hospitalization is not appropriate for the majority of dementia patients. Short-term and (later) long-term assisted care are much more readily available, and both can be administered either in the patient's home or elsewhere. We discuss both here, and we give special emphasis to the best known form of long-term care, the nursing home.

Extended Care

Let us look first at three kinds of hospitals and describe the role that each can play in the care of persons suffering from a dementing illness. These are state hospitals, VA hospitals, and private hospitals.

State Hospitals

State hospitals provide care for mentally ill persons, and until recently these facilities were used mainly for long-term custody. But today, few people suffering from dementia are found in state hospitals. A few are there because their behavior is too disruptive or dangerous for nursing homes to manage. But state hospitals became less import after Medicaid began funding nursing home care in 1965. However, in order to qualify for Medicaid benefits, most people must also qualify for SSI benefits. (Supplemental Security Income is a federal program that guarantees for low income elderly persons, and the disabled, a minimum income sufficent to pay for care in a nursing home.) It is those who cannot qualify for SSI who may need state hospitals.

In spite of the bad reputations that many people associate with them, state hospitals are not places to be feared. The better ones have complete nursing staffs and offer many of the same services as private hospitals, including occupational, physical, and recreational therapy. Most are self-contained and have laboratories, x-ray equipment, and special units for patients with physical problems. Social workers and members of the nursing staff are available to work with families. Most staff members are caring people devoted to their patients.

Subject to their meeting certain requirements, state hospitals are eligible to be paid through Medicare benefits. The hospital must be accredited and must provide active treatment. Because of the limited coverage in Medicare and private insurance programs, the patient or relatives must assume some of the cost for care in a state hospital, if they are able to do so. The amount is based on annual gross income and household size. If the family is unable to pay, the state hospital will provide care regardless.

Admission to a state hospital may be voluntary or by judicial commitment. Information about commitment and admission procedures can be obtained from social service departments at county court offices. Visit your state hospitals. In some states you may find them to be badly run, poorly maintained institutions. But you are much more likely to be pleasantly surprised with the caring staff and the variety of opportunities available to patients.

Just as only a small proportion of dementia patients live in state hospitals, care in VA hospitals is limited to another subset of the population of dementia victims.

Veterans Administration Hospitals

If the person with dementia is a veteran, it is worthwhile to contact your nearest Veterans Administration Medical Center (hospital) to learn about the services it offers. The Veterans

Administration operates some of the largest health care facilities in the United States. Many are affiliated with university medical schools. All offer a wide range of services to veterans who qualify. Each Veterans Administration Medical Center offers specific programs and services that vary with the resources available, but the VA hospital's first priority is to care for veterans whose disabilities or medical problems are service-related. In addition, budgetary constraints have forced the VA medical system to restrict eligibility among those whose conditions are not service-connected to low-income veterans who cannot finance their own care. For example, single veterans seeking care at a VA hospital for a non-service-connected illness or disability must have resources (income and liquid assets) totaling less than $22,000. "Liquid assets" exclude the veteran's home, home furnishings, and automobiles, but the formulas are complex; see a VA consultant.

In addition to their general program, the Veterans Administration medical system has developed special centers— Geriatric Research, Education, and Clinical Centers (GRECCs)—dedicated to research and education in the aging processes and associated disease. Each of the thirteen centers in the GRECC system has a specific area of interest, and each recruits the expert researchers and clinicians it needs to focus on that particular aspect of aging. Some of the areas being studied are cardiology, neurology, psychiatry, immunology, nutrition, diabetes and other diseases of metabolism, dementia, and aspects of general medicine. GRECCs are located at the following Veterans Administration Medical Centers:

- Arkansas
  Little Rock

- California
  Los Angeles (Wadsworth)
  Palo Alto
  Sepulveda

- Florida
  Gainesville

o Massachusetts
  Boston (Brockton/West Roxbury Division)

o Michigan
  Ann Arbor

o Minnesota
  Minneapolis

o Missouri
  St. Louis

o North Carolina
  Durham

o Texas
  San Antonio

o Washington
  Seattle
  American Lake

Some GRECCs offer special programs and services that can be helpful to veterans with dementia. We suggest that when contacting a Veterans Administration Medical Center in one of the foregoing cities, you start by asking to talk to someone in the GRECC program. If that GRECC is unable to meet the needs of the veteran with dementia or suspected dementia, the medical team can make informed referrals to other VA hospitals or community resources.

We have seen that both state and VA hospitals tend to be appropriate settings only for early dementia patient who have quite special needs or qualifications. In the next section we shall see how the role of the private hospital in the care of a dementia patient is more limited still.

Private Hospitals

Private hospitals offer medical care, clinical evaluation, and social service support for families, but most do not offer extended nursing care for victims of dementia—the cost would be

prohibitive for all but the wealthiest families. However, these
hospitals often receive patients with an acute illness and,
before that illness is controlled, find themselves in the position
of making the first evaluation of an apparent dementia. When
dementia is known to be present, it helps if a family member
explains the patient's behavior and routine to the professional
staff. Hospital personnel are usually aware of the kinds of
problems persons with dementia face. However, for their own
understanding it is important for family members to ask the
following questions.

- Is the patient going to be placed in an open or a locked
  area?

- Is there adequate nursing staff during the night?

- What diagnostic testing will be done and when?

As is true in any hospitalization, families should leave
their names and the telephone numbers at which they can be
reached if problems arise.

Private hospitals usually have social service departments
that are valuable resources for counseling and information.
Social workers help with financial and home care planning, and
they know what services are available in the community.

For example, social workers can generally help with the
rental or purchase of equipment needed for home care and can
supply information about a wide variety of things, including
visiting nurses, transportation, medical care, insurance
coverage, and pensions. Social workers also assist with place-
ments in nursing homes. They know what local nursing home
facilities have to offer and keep lists of available vacancies.

Alternatives to Early Nursing Home Care

Nursing home placement was once the only alternative for most
families when caring at home for a person with dementia
became overwhelming. However, alternatives to nursing
homes now exist, and some families feel that they can provide

better care for their loved one at home with supplemental help. Hence they choose to delay as long as practical the time when they will have to pay the high cost of nursing home care.

Respite Care

Respite care describes various forms of help available to families. Respite care can consist of adult day care, in-home help with caring for the patient, or short-term residential care at an overnight facility. We will briefly examine all of these alternatives.

Respite care is a service organization's intermittent assumption of responsibility for the ill person. Thus it frees the primary caregiver for a specified period of time. When such temporary relief is available, caregivers often find that they are able to cope longer with the demands of caring for their loved one at home. Respite care is usually provided by a nonprofessional who has had some special training either through a program sponsored by an Alzheimer's Association chapter or through a university. Respite care can be provided in the home or at hospitals, nursing homes, churches, day care centers, or senior citizen complexes. (Several forms of respite care are offered in most large metropolitan areas, whereas in rural communities, this alternative may not be available.) Centers differ in the services they offer. Some provide respite care during the day while the caregiver works; others may offer only four or six hours per week—enough time to give the homebound caregiver a chance to shop or visit with friends. Many of these programs, although they may be affiliated with a university or an Alzheimer's Association chapter, are not monitored or licensed. It is wise to do some checking before enrolling a family member.

Day Care

Adult day care has become popular in recent years. Most of the orginal adult day care facilites were designed to serve persons whose mental impairment is minimal, but programs specifically designed for confused persons have become available in many areas. Day care centers offer limited nursing care, but the emphasis is on keeping those attending active as long as possible. The family of the dementia patient can avail itself of these facilities daily or only a few times per week or month (but bear in mind that the value, to the patient, of familiar surroundings is enhanced by regular visits). There are also "night" care centers in some areas to give the tired caregiver a chance to sleep. The programs are run by paid staff or volunteers and are usually associated with a church or hospital. The cost of day care can vary widely and is often based on a sliding scale, which means that charges are adjusted according to ability to pay. Fees range from $10 to $70 per day.

Timing is crucial when you are planning to enlist the services of a day care center. Persons with dementia should be introduced to the new environment early enough in the course of the illness to be able to make the adjustment and become comfortable with the staff and setting. If placement is left until the later stages of the illness, the person with dementia may not adjust. Be aware, however, that some persons in the early stages of the illness have difficulty adjusting to the day care situation because they are functioning at a relatively high level and become upset upon seeing others who are more severely impaired.

When choosing a day care center, it is most important to select one that can meet the needs of individuals at different stages of dementing illness. The day care staff should be warm, friendly, and (most important) patient. Social workers should be available to help the patient and family work through some of the frustrations of everyday living. A separate room, away from the group, is desirable where individuals can be alone with a staff person should they get upset. Provisions should be made to curb wandering. An active, stilmulating environment with a low patient-to-staff ratio is essential. Time spent in a day care enter will not slow the progression of Alzheimer's disease, but it can provide pleasure for the ill person and can offer vital respite to the caregiver.

Respite Care in the Home

In-home respite care can be arranged through health care agencies or through those Alzheimer's Association chapters that have special respite care projects. Because in-home respite caregivers are nonprofessionals, a careful evaluation of the services required and the needs of the ill person should be made. A good first step in hiring an in-home respite helper is to contact people who have had a similar experience and can recommend agencies or individuals who understand the illness and the special care needed. Before allowing a helper into the home, families chould check that helper's references carefully.

Another variety of in-home care is offered through the ACTION Senior Companion Program in which some local chapters of the Alzheimer's Association are currently participating. (Contact the local Alzheimer's Association chapter for additional information, or check under "health care agencies" in the yellow pages of the telephone directory). This program offers respite for the caregiver but does not provide the nursing skills some families need. Alzheimer's Association chapters identify families that may benefit from this type of respite, and some chapters conduct ongoing training sessions for the home care helpers. Companions are compensated volunteers who receive a stipend and are reimbursed for expenses. These helpers are nonprofessionals and may not be able to handle some complex needs, but they do give the caregiver time off. Because this service is monitored by Alzheimer's Association chapters, primary caregivers can feel confident that the companion is trustworthy and has had special training. There is a charge for this service, and only limited financial assistance is available. However, many projects are partly supported through hospitals, grants, or private foundations.

Residential Respite Care Away from Home

Another source of respite for families is offered by hospitals, nursing homes, and some Alzheimer's Association chapters. Sometimes residential care outside the home for a few days or weeks is needed when an emergency such as illness of the primary caregiver arises. It is also available to caregivers who need vacation time.

Residental respite offers weekend and overnights stays. Except that some programs will not accept patients who wander, it is available for persons in the advanced stages of the disease. An important benefit derived from complete respite is that it may help caregivers realize how difficult home care has become. Sometimes having availed themselves of residential respite care makes it easier for families to decide that the time has come to arrange for long-term care in a nursing home facility.

And for all patients with dementia who do not succumb to another illness, that time eventually comes. The rest of this chapter is devoted to discussing long-term care: alternative settings, criteria to use in evaluating nursing homes, and means of financing nursing home care.

Long-Term Care

When the caregiver can no longer manage without full-time assistance, long-term care, either in a care facility or at home, becomes necessary. Long-term care is defined as assistance, over an indefinite period, with everyday activities such as eating, bathing, and getting dressed. Long-term care does not usually involve constant medical attention, and it can be given at home, in the community, or in an institution.

Long-Term Nursing Care at Home

Many products, and several services, are available to help ill and disabled people preserve some independence and to help their families continue working and living much as they did before the disability began. Local social service agencies and your chapter of the Alzheimer's Association have the names of organizations that help with home nursing care. Community and fraternal organizations may rent equipment such as hospital beds, wheelchairs, and walkers. Others provide transportation. "Meals on Wheels" delivers one hot meal a day to people who cannot cook for themselves.

Sooner or later, however, the time comes when someone must stay at home with a person who suffers from dementia. The spouse may choose early retirement from work in order to provide needed care and to minimize nursing and custodial costs. There are many trade-offs to consider in this decision. Early retirement reduces the years available to work and build up entitlement to full retirement benefits. The able partner must also give up the friendship of coworkers and the stimulation that comes from a job. Eventually, too, the disabled person will require nursing home care, leaving the able family member or spouse with a reduced retirement income and the need to develop new relationships and to renew old interests.

These and other drawbacks, such as the physically demanding nature of some of the care the loved one needs, may tempt the family to bring someone else in to provide long-term care at home. We are convinced, however, that hiring someone to give nursing care in the home does not work well unless exceptional help is available. It is extremely difficult to hire dependable caregivers. Furthermore, provision has to be made for days off, vacations,and sick days. There are agencies that will provide nursing help (at the aide level) for about $75.00 for two shifts, but our experience suggests that the quality of care provided is not high. If you choose this alternative be alert for any sign of neglect or even abuse of the patient. Expect to try out and discharge several persons before finding two or three who are responsible. And expect to have to take over regularly on short notice, because someone does not show up for work.

Skilled-Nursing Homes

Skilled-nursing homes provide 24-hour nursing care and also offer rehabilitation services. A home such as this is the clear choice for people who are convalescing or who have a long-term illness. Nursing care is provided by a staff of registered and licensed practical nurses, who can administer medications and implement procedures ordered by physicians. Physical and occupational therapy are emphasized, and trained therapists work with doctors to develop specific plans for meeting individuals' needs.

A skilled-nursing home may be part of a medical complex, or it may be a separate facility. After the acute-care hospital, it is the most expensive alternative. The cost varies between $70 and $100 per day ($2100 to $3000 per month). Check with your local health care association, Alzheimer's Association chapter, or health care ombudsman for recommendations and costs for your area. If family resources permit, the patient may enter a skilled-nursing home as a private-pay resident. Medicare and most health care insurance policies do not cover nursing home costs, and nursing home insurance (policies specifically designed to cover such care) are costly. Their coverage is also quite limited.

How to Evaluate a Nursing Home

When choosing a nursing home, visit several homes suggested by your local Alzheimer' Association chapter or social service agency. It is wise to visit unannounced in order to have an opportunity to evaluate the normal operations of the home. Sometimes first impressions may be the best guide: What are your first impressions upon entering the nursing home? Is there a disagreeable odor? If a number of patients are sitting together in one large room, are they talking to one another? Are staff members circulating among the residents, or are they in the nursing station chatting over coffee? Do some residents have smiles on their faces, or are all staring off into space or sleeping? How many nurses are interacting with patients? Do you see staff members in individual rooms or walking with patients in the halls? Does the nursing staff refer to the patients as Mr., Miss, or Mrs. or by their first names? (The former is generally a reliable sign that respect is accorded the resident and that they are not being condescended to). What are your impressions when you visit the dining room and the activity room where the residents watch television?

Now do some research: What is the patient-to-staff ratio? Are medical consultants and physical and recreational therapists available? Are regular staff meetings scheduled with families? Ask about the staff. Are the nurses registered nurses or practical nurses? Are both types on duty both day and night? How are nurses' aides trained, and what is the ratio of patients to social workers? Does the nursing home have a current state license? Has the home been inspected by the state? Do the members of the administrative staff hold current licenses? If you anticipate asking for Medicaid assistance, inquire whether the home is approved for payments from Medicaid and whether it accepts "Medicaid patients"?

Note the physical conditions and atmosphere: Are all areas well lighted? Are there handrails in the hallways and grab bars in the bathrooms? Is the furniture sturdy? Does the home meet federal and state fire codes? Are doors to stairways kept closed, and is there an emergency evacuation plan? Do staff members and patients practice fire drills regularly? (No one likes to think of a loved one roused from sleep and upset by a fire drill. At the same time, no one likes to think of a loved one dying in flames because staff members and patients had never practiced the evacuation plan. Fire drills are obviously the lesser evil).

Take note of the residents' bedrooms: Are they pleasant and clean? Do all rooms open onto a hall, and is there a window in each room? How many residents are in a room? Is there a closet or large locker for each resident? Does each bed have a bell for calling the nurse and a drape that can be drawn for privacy? Are the rooms decorated with bright colors, curtains, and attractive furniture? How close is the nursing staff to the residents' bedrooms? Is there a lounge that can be used for family visits or parties?

Observe the dining room: Is it attractive? Are there windows? Are the residents talking to one another? Are the meals served at the table or cafeteria style, and by whom—staff or patients? Does the food look appetizing? Sample some. Are patients who need help with eating continously assisted? Is the kitchen clean and well equipped? Are sanitation rules posted and observed by kitchen workers?

Investigate the medical and other services available: Is the patient's personal physician allowed to order prescriptions and write orders in the patient's chart. What medical records are kept? Are patients' activities charted on a daily basis? Other than medical services, what professional services are available? Is there a dentist or optometrist on the staff? How does the nursing home deal with medical emergencies? How close is the nearest hospital, and what plan is in place to provide transportation to it if the need should arise?

Inquire about programs available for residents: Is a physical therapist on duty, and are any specific therapies requested by the patients' physicians available? If a recreational therapist is on the staff, are there some activities geared to the declining capabilities typical of the dementing patient? How are volunteers used? For example, do they give nursing care or assist in group activities? Are members of the clergy available? Are barbers and beauticians on location, or are patients transported for these services?

After you have chosen a nursing home to meet the patient's needs and the family's standards, it is time to turn your attention to cost. Cost is an important issue because nursing home care can range from $70 to $100 per day. Families should meet with administrators and social workers to discuss financial arrangements in detail. All financial agreements should be in writing, and copies should be given to family members.

It is time for us, also, to turn our attention to costs and review some of the sources of financial help available for long-term care of victims of dementia.

Family Financial Resources and Long-Term Care

Many families need help with the financial burdens imposed by dementia. If the nursing home has been certified by Medicare,* there may be some financial help for the patient.

---

* Most nursing homes in the United States are not skilled-nursing facilities and hence are not eligible for Medicare certification. Furthermore, even many skilled-nursing facilities are not certified by Medicare.

When skilled nursing care is needed, all services for the first 20 days are paid by Medicare. After the first 20 days, Medicare pays a portion of the daily rate for the next 80 days. Then other arrangements must be made. This is because, unfortunately, persons who have a dementing illness are assumed to require only custodial care. In order to receive Medicare benefits, patients' have to be classified as "needing medically skilled nursing care." Medicare may cover some skilled nursing care when that care is provided in a traditional nursing home or as home health care, but the eligibility rules are very strict. It is safest to assume you will not be able to rely on Medicare.

Medical Assistance (Medicaid)

When family resources are limited, medical assistance (Medicaid), a combination of federal and state financial aid administered by counties, can help to cover the cost. In order for a patient to receive Medicaid assistance, the patient's resources (assets plus income) must not exceed an established low amount. To be eligible patients must "spend down" their resources to the required level. In the past this provision meant impoverishment for the spouse who continued to live in the community.

However, a "spousal impoverishment" portion of the Medicare Catastrophic Coverage Act of 1988 eases that burden somewhat. The act established nationwide guidelines for protection of the financial resources of spouses of patients who need nursing home care. It includes the division of assets between spouses and assurance of income for the well spouse. Check with your county welfare department for more information about of Medicaid and about how it may apply in your specific situation.

Private Long-Term Care Insurance

Whether private long-term care insurance ("nursing home insurance") can protect American families against the catastrophic cost of long-term care or whether, alternatively, a universal, public insurance program is needed, is being debated at this time.

Most nursing home insurance policies could be viewed as asset protection, not health insurance. The insurance is designed to cover some of the costs of nursing home care, thus protecting family assets from the "spending down" involved in establishing eligibility for Medicaid. But unless there are assets worth more than $50,000 (not including home and automobile) an annual income of more than $10,000 or dependents or others to whom the victim of dementia and his or her spouse wish to leave an estate, this type of insurance may not be appropriate. In addition, policies are not issued for "preexisting conditions," so benefits are not available to a person with dementia unless the policy was taken out before the onset of the disease.

Premiums on long-term care insurance can range from $600 to more than $2000 a year, depending on the level of daily benefits chosen. The higher the daily benefit, the higher the premium. Bear in mind that nursing home rates are rising and that few policies make any provision for inflation. Some states have established regulations to make sure that Alzheimer's disease and other dementias are not excluded from coverage. Should you decide to purchase a nursing home policy, compare the costs and benefits of several different insurance plans, ask to see a specimen policy that illustrates exactly what is covered, and don't allow yourself to be pressured. Be sure that

- The insurance company is financially sound, having earned an A. M. Best rating of A+ or A.

- Alzheimer's disease or dementia is covered and not specifically excluded from coverage.

- There is no requirement that the patient be hospitalized before qualifying for nursing home benefits.

- There is no requirement that the patient have needed prior skilled nursing care before qualifying for intermediate or custodial care.

Many senior citizen organizations provide literature that can help families decide whether to buy long-term care insurance. If you decide to do so, be sure to read your policy carefully when you receive it; within 30 days from that time you have the right to cancel it and receive a refund.

Other sources of financial help include Social Security, Aid to Families with Dependent Children, disability income, Supplemental Security Income, veterans' benefits, and private health insurance, which will, cover at least the diagnostic costs associated with dementia. Many resources are intended to provide primarily crisis-oriented, short-term care and are therefore perceived as not being appropriate for victims of Alzheimer's disease who require long-term care. Only through systematic exploration can you collect all the facts you will need to determine what aid you are eligible for and what care alternatives you can afford.

8

Practical Matters

Much of the material in this chapter is practical knowledge: What to tell children, relatives, and neighbors; what legal rights and responsibilites are involved; what help to expect from insurance, retirement plans, and Social Security. Because every situation is unique, only general guidelines can be presented. States offer different services and each has its own laws, so legal issues are especially complex. Consulting state-level social service departments or a local chapter of the Alzheimer's Association may be the best way to become familiar with local resources. Most families need an attorney who is well versed in the laws and regulations that govern financing long-term care, preserving assets, and legal competency.

Dealing with Children, Relatives, and Neighbors

Children in the Home

Children living in a household where a person is showing signs of dementia are always aware of the changes and realize that a problem exists. But children usually do not know how to react to the situation. Sometimes they understand only the effect it has on them and on other family members.

The parent's best course is to be truthful with children mature enough to understand and to tell them exactly what is happening. The problem that is, or soon will be, affecting the entire family cannot be hidden or covered up. Parents should also tell their children what the doctors have said is likely to happen and, should, if possible, make an appointment for the children to see one of the doctors to ask questions. In the long run, they will be better able to accept the person with dementia and the effects of the disease if they know the basic facts.

Indeed, children sometimes cope with a nonfunctioning parent or grandparent better than adults do. Children often make fewer demands than adults. They don't converse on abstract topics. Like all of us, children (especially teenagers), can become angry and frustrated at the failures of the ill person, and they may find it difficult to understand the lack of interest such persons often have in the child or grandchild's world. Yet, in general, children do very well with mentally incompetent adults. They may actually assume a parental role by telling their ill parent or grandparent what to do and when to do it, and by reacting effectively in situations where judgment is required. Children quickly learn the "do's and don'ts" of handling the parent or grandparent who suffers from dementia. And if the affected individual gets into a potentially dangerous situation, children are generally quick to step in and protect him or her from possible harm.

A special problem for many children is embarrassment in front of their friends. They may not want friends to visit the home because they are afraid that the ill person will do or say something strange. Concerned about what other kids will think, some children choose not to tell their friends. Others do tell friends and classmates and share information about the disease, much to the benefit of all concerned. Parents should not push children on this matter, however. Encourage them to talk freely about any problems they encounter, and give them time to learn to cope with the situation in their own way. The Alzheimer's Association has brochures, books, and videotapes to help children and teenagers understand and cope. Some Alzheimer's Association chapters even have special support groups for teenagers.

Placing a parent or grandparent in a nursing home, or just deciding upon nursing home placement, is hard for the entire family. When the time does come and placement has been made, the caregiving family feels a sense of loss mixed with relief. This reaction is normal. Though children may be particularly affected by the loss; they usually quickly resume their regular pattern of living.

Parents often have trouble accepting it when children say they do not want to visit the nursing home. Children should not be made to feel guilty or pushed into making visits. Give the children time, and they will make the right decision. When children choose to go with the family for a visit, the visit should be kept short because the parent or grandparent's progressive deterioration can upset the child. Many children do develop a sense of deepened understanding and compassion through visiting a relative in a nursing home. We advise against younger children visiting after the condition has worsened to the point where the ill person does not recognize visitors.

What to Tell Relatives and Neighbors

Be truthful with everyone in the family, even if it is difficult. A spouse or child who must explain the diagnosis to relatives usually encounters one of two reactions. Either the family is very supportive of the spouse (or other family member) who is providing the care and understands the situation, or the family refuses to accept the fact that something is wrong with the ill person. Some relatives blame the situation on other circumstances: "You have made mother unhappy." " You must not have fed dad properly." "If you had been more attentive, this would never have happened." Sometimes family members choose to attribute what is happening to normal aging: "He's just getting old."

At the time when families are first faced with a diagnosis of dementia, social support for the prospective care giver is essential. Talking with family members and friends and sharing concerns about the future can be extremely helpful. Attending an Alzheimer's Association support group meeting, wherein members of other affected families share their experience, can be useful. Obtaining as much educational material as possible is also important. We have found that families who are well informed about the future are better able to handle problems that arise.

Even caregivers who have the support of other family members may sometimes feel they have not done all that is possible. Continued reassurance is important, which is one reason why information about the patient should be shared. Accounts of doctor's visits, consultations with specialists, hospital evaluations, and daily happenings should be circulated among all family members.

To give other family members some idea of how demanding the caregiver's job is, ask them to care for the patient for a few days while the caregiver gets some rest. That experience will help them understand why the primary caregiver has made certain choices. Share the literature that is available with all family members, and invite them to attend an Alzheimer's Association support group meeting where they can ask questions and visit with others who are dealing with the same kinds of problems.

Even when a family tries to keep the ill person hidden indoors, neighbors are well aware that something is wrong. (All that is really "wrong," of course, is acting as though the illness were something to be ashamed of and keeping neighbors in the dark.) Be truthful. Tell the neighbors exactly what has happened. Also, give them information about the illness so they will not be afraid of the behaviors they may observe and will be better prepared to handle a difficult situation if one should arise. Share with them brochures available from the Alzheimer's Association that discuss the disease, its symptoms, and home care of the victim.

Families most often find that neighbors are thoughtful and help a great deal. They call when they see the patient wandering about or doing something dangerous. They provide moral support to the caregiver by visiting. And they can be there at a moment's notice if the situation should become difficult to control.

Competence and Legal Responsibility

Difficulty in maintaining financial records is often an indicator of the early stages of dementia. More than the usual number of checks may be incorrectly recorded, or several may have been written and not recorded at all. Problems with simple addition and subtraction are common.

Families may also find that unwise financial decisions have been made. Sometimes these decisions have long-term effects on the family's financial situation. The affected person may have sold property, for example, or given away jewelry, furs, or other expensive personal items.

Thus it is important for family members to gather all financial documents together, in the early stages of the illness, and assess the family's financial status. They should review savings and investment accounts and throughly understand the assets and financial commitments involved. This is important, because within a short period of time the person affected may become unable to provide a coherent history of financial transactions, let alone manage them.

Efforts to ease the legal and financial responsibilities of a person in the early stages of dementia may be met by hostility. The ill person may become overly suspicious and mistrustful, telling friends and neighbors that the family is stealing, or may even call the police to ask for help. If resistance does develop, it may be passive, and family members may be able to assume enough authority to exercise *de facto* control. Often, however, they have no choice but to obtain legal control; bills must be paid and family assets need to be protected. In general, hostility based on loss of financial authority is short-lived. Those suffering from dementia may even be grateful to be relieved of the anxiety they feel when tackling mental tasks that they can no longer manage.

No matter what the course of the disease, at some point the ill person will no longer be capable of making financial decisions. If this person has been the main wage earner and has handled the family's financial affairs, the spouse (or someone designated by the family) will have to assume the responsibility. Legal assistance will be required.

Legal action through the courts may be required in order to empower a spouse or other family member to act on behalf of an ill person. This is true even when the ill individual cannot understand what is happening or has become physically unable to sign documents. This authority is usually acquired through a conservatorship, a power of attorney, or a guardianship. In considering any of these legal procedures, it is well to remember that a declaration of incompetence is a legal judgment rendered by a court.

CONSERVATORSHIP A conservatorship is set up by an individual to protect, guide, and maintain his or her financial affairs. If dementia is in its early stages, the individual affected may appoint another person or financial agency to act in his or her behalf through a conservatorship. Some people realize that they are losing their ability to manage financially and initiate this process themselves. However, when it is determined that the person with dementia is no longer capable of managing assets, a petition to establish a conservatorship can be filed by a family member or close friend. Other family members receive notice of the petition and can contest it if they choose. A conservatorship is granted by a court and remains under the supervision of the courts.

POWER OF ATTORNEY A power of attorney is a written statement legally authorizing one person, the attorney-in-fact, to act on behalf of another. In addition to financial management, a power of attorney conveys the authority to buy and sell real estate and to manage property. Whether limited or general in scope, the power of attorney, however, is likely to be useful only in the early stages of dementia, because for it to remain in force, the person who gives it must know what is being done.

DURABLE POWER OF ATTORNEY This type of document remains in effect even after the ill person is no longer legally competent. Thus it is more effective than the simple power of attorney in addressing the need for help in managing financial affairs and health care that people with dementia eventually have. A durable power of attorney must be signed by a person who is still capable and of sound mind; its real benefit for victims of dementia and their families is that it remains in force for the rest of the patient's life. It can stipulate guidelines that the attorney-in-fact must follow and can include authority decisions about health care. The attorney-in-fact is legally responsible for making decisions that are in the best interest of the person with dementia.

GUARDIANSHIP Establishment of a guardianship is a legal process that results in the appointment of an individual or agency to handle the affairs of a person who can no longer function independently. The guardian appointed by the count can be a family member, some other individual (such as a lawyer) or an institution. The guardian must protect and care for the person and property of one who is found incapable of managing her or his own affairs. A family member can usually initiate this process, but the court maintains supervisory rights over the guardian or institution appointed.

INCOME TAX Even the simple process of filling out joint income tax returns may become complicated if one partner cannot sign the form. In such a case, the family should obtain a special power-of-attorney tax form, which gives specific authority to act for another person in all matters pertaining to taxes. This form is available at any branch office of the Internal Revenue Service and at state tax offices. Consult your tax advisor about any other tax concerns, such as the possible advantages of minimizing estate taxes by giving gifts and establishing trusts while the victim is still competent.

PROPERTY The spouse must consider joint ownership of property. In most cases, joint ownership is a great advantage because the property is in both names, and therefore, in most instances, the able partner can take over ownership. In some cases, however, it may be preferable to transfer the title to certain properties, including those jointly owned, to the well spouse, another family member, or a trusted friend. Some state laws protect the interest of an ill spouse in property, regardless of who holds the title.

When nursing home care is required, liquid assets that are still in the patient's name (with certain exceptions; see Chapter 7) must be used to pay for care in that home before the patient is eligible for Medicaid assistance. Sometimes young dependents are involved; their care should be considered when planning for the future. An attorney may be able to help families find ways to conserve assets for their needs. The best advice to any family is to consult an attorney who has some knowledge of dementing disease and is familiar with current regulations governing eligibility for assistance in financing long-term care.

Insurance and Insurability

Health Care Insurance

Health care insurance coverage for persons who become disabled, including those with dementia, is a major concern. Most of us do not think about health insurance benefits or coverage until we need them.

When families are faced with illness and have little or no health insurance coverage, they may panic. They may, on impulse, buy any policy they can get—and regret their haste when they try to use it.

Employed persons are usually insured by a company group health care plan. If they should become disabled and cannot work, that insurance coverage generally remains in force for one additional year. After that, they may have the option of converting the policy and paying the premiums themselves. But in most cases, converting from a group policy to individual or family coverage is costly; many can not afford it. If there is a company-sponsored disability program, it may pay for continued health and life insurance benefits (see discussion in next section on Disability).

Those who cannot pay for insurance coverage may apply for county assistance. If they are fortunate enough to live in a state that provides a comprehensive health care plan, they may be covered under this type of insurance. However, there is generally a six-month waiting period before a comprehensive health care policy provides benefits.

Most health insurance policies contain a clause stating that any preexisting illness, such as progressive dementia, is not covered. After the diagnosis is made and recorded in Medicare records, the ill person is for all practical purposes no longer insurable. State health plans, however, cannot include a clause exempting preexisting illnesses, so this may be a source of financial help. Unfortunately, state health plans do not exist in all states. Families should check with their local insurance board to find out what options for health care coverage are available in the state where they live.

Health Maintenance Organizations (HMOs)

Health maintenance organizations may be a source of help for people who receive Medicare benefits. The Health Care Financing Administration, which administers HMOs, also administers the Medicare program and encourages Medicare beneficiaries to consider joining an HMO that has a Medicare contract. Many services offered by such an HMO are covered by Medicare. And most HMOs offer other services for an additional premium.

Like an insurance company, an HMO pays the costs of health care (including both physicians' charges and hospital bills) for a monthly premium. There are two types of HMOs: those operating from one central location and those operating from the offices of individual doctors. The advantages of joining an HMO include availability of all services needed, such as doctors' services, hospital care, laboratory tests, x-rays, and emergency care. Those who use the service of an HMO must continue to pay the monthly Medicare medical insurance (Medicare Part B). For most people this premium is deducted from their monthly Social Security check. Medicare interprets the premium paid to an HMO as paid to a co-insurer and therefore counts it against deductibles.

Medicare benefits, which include medical costs, are available for persons who are disabled (unable to work and under age 65) and who have been receiving disability checks from Social Security for two years. These benefits provide hospital insurance protection at no charge to the individual; however, participants who want insurance covering physicians' services and medication must pay a monthly premium.

Life Insurance

If the patient is under age 65 and a diagnosis of Alzheimer's disease has been made, life insurance policies on that person's life should be checked to see whether they contain provisions granting disability waivers of premium. Sixty-five is the age at which disability ends and retirement begins. These waivers cover the cost of premiums when the insured is designated as disabled. This type of coverage is usually offered at very low additional cost, on life insurance (and often on mortgage insurance) at the time when employment begins or the policy is issued. Insurance policies differ, however, and the definition of *disabled* can vary from "unable to do certain kinds of work" to "unable ever to work again." When a diagnosis of dementia is made at an early age, disability insurance premium waivers can save the family money and make it possible for them to keep life insurance policies in force.

Disability and Retirement Plans

Many employers provide retirement plans to supplement their employees' incomes in the retirement years. Once employees have worked the minimum number of years required by the plan, they are entitled to benefits when they reach retirement age. If the person with dementia is over sixty-five, has already retired, and is receiving benefits at the time of diagnosis, no change occurs in those benefits.

Usually, people who choose to retire at an early age receive benefits at a reduced rate. Although people are eligible for retirement at age 62 or younger, full benefits are usually based on retirement at age 65. When people apply for Social Security benefits before they are 65, their monthly payment is reduced by an amount that depends on the number of monthly checks they will receive before they reach age 65.

When a person must stop working early because of illness (such as dementia), however, a disability exists. If the employee was a participant in a company disability plan, benefits should be claimed under that plan. Most disability insurance plans are coordinated with Social Security disability benefits and guarantee an income that is a certain percentage of the worker's wages at the time of disablement. For example, if a person earned $3000 a month and the disability plan guaranteed 60 percent of that income should a participant become disabled, Social Security would pay a portion according to the Social Security scale, and the insurance would make up the difference up to 60 percent of $3000, or $1800 a month. These benefits may include hospitalization and life insurance.

After applying for any existing disability insurance benefits, the family should apply for disability payments to the person with dementia under Social Security disability. (Guidelines by which eligibility for disability benefits are determined are discussed in the next section). Because of the long-term effects of dementing illness, victims of this disease are better off financially if they apply for benefits as early as possible.

Social Security and Other Government Programs

Social Security Retirement/Disability

Social Security provides a continuing income when family earnings are reduced or ended because of retirement, disability, or death. This program is nearly always available to families of persons with dementing illness.

To be eligible to receive cash benefits, one must have done at least a minimum amount of work under Social Security. Social Security credit is measured in quarters of coverage; there are four quarters of coverage for each year. The exact amount of work credit depends on one's age and on the quarter in which coverage began. People who stop working under Social Security before they have worked enough quarters are not eligible to receive benefits.

However, work credit for disability benefits is different if a person becomes disabled at age 31 or later. For persons 31 years old or older, the requirement for eligibility is only five years of work credit out of the ten years prior to the onset of disability.

Under Social Security guidelines, a person is considered disabled when a physical or mental condition exists that prevents him or her from doing substantial work and when the condition is expected to last, or has lasted, for twelve months or is likely to result in death. Applicants must provide medical evidence of the severity of the condition and must prove that the condition prevents their working.

Persons who are receiving disability benefits can also receive money for children who are unmarried and under 18 years old or who are unmarried and attend high school full time. A spouse 62 years old or older is also eligible.

Disability benefits begin after five months. Because no benefits are paid for those first five months, disability must exist for a full six months before the first payment can be received. Apply for benefits as soon as possible after disability is established. Back payments are limited to the twelve months preceding the month during which application was made.

Supplemental Security Income (SSI)

Another federal program, Supplemental Security Income (SSI), is operated for the benefit of persons who are disabled or who have little or no income or resources. This program provides benefits even when income is available from other sources, including Social Security.

Although the Social Security Administration administers SSI, it is not the same as Social Security. SSI payments come from the general funds of the U.S. Treasury, whereas Social Security benefits are drawn from contributions made by workers, employers, and self-employed persons.

Under the Supplemental Security Income program, state, federal, and local governments work together, but the federal government administers this program through the Social Security Administration. States supplement federal payments by providing Medicaid, food stamps, and social rehabilitation.

The financial assistance offered by SSI is relatively free of restrictions. Those who receive this assistance can keep their home, and there is no lien requirement. Personal property, including an automobile of reasonable value, can also be retained.

For patients in institutions, there are three exceptions to the rules concerning eligibility for SSI payments;

1. SSI payments may be denied if the recipient resides in a public or private health care facility that is receiving payments from Medicaid.

2. The payment may be reduced if the recipient is living in a publicly operated community residence that serves no more than 16 people.

3. The patient may not be eligible if she or he is staying in a public institutuion primarily in order to get approved education or vocational training.

Those who are receiving SSI must apply for any other financial benefits that may be due them under Social Security. If those other benefits are received, SSI payments can be reduced. However, the state may augment SSI payments without penalty if the state's payment is made regularly and is based on need.

Contact any Social Security office for additional information about Social Security benefits, Medicare, or SSI. Look in the phone directory under U.S. Government Offices and/or Social Security Administration, or ask for information at a U.S. Post Office.

Ethical Decisions

Family members, caregivers, guardians, and conservators often find themselves involved in crucial treatment decisions. Whether to see that heroic measures are undertaken to resuscitate a person with dementia whose illness is well advanced, for example, and whether to treat vigorously other illnesses that may develop in such individuals, are decisions that are hard for family members, professional caregivers, and doctors to make. The fact that the patient is unable to share in such decisions makes the situation even more difficult.

Of course, victims of Alzheimer's disease and related dementias also come from different cultural and religious backgrounds, and these factors cannot be overlooked. Sometimes religious counselors or members of the clergy are involved in family discussions. In addition, some doctors and nurses have strong feelings about what care should—and should not—be offered to patients in the final stages of any disease.

The Alzheimer's Association has issued guidelines for the treatment of patients with advanced dementia that may prove helpful to families and physicians facing these issues. Any private or government hospital can explain its policy on do-not-resuscitate (DNR) orders for persons in the last stages of an illness,and most can provide an ethics counselor for families who wish to solicit his or her advice.

Decisions about whether to prolong life, and whether to prolong dying, are easier for all if a living will has been executed and its signing witnessed. A growing number of states have passed legislation that provides a vehicle for people to indicate their desires in this regard while they are still competent to do so. In the living will, a proxy can be named to make decisions on behalf of the person completing the document. Families should discuss this key concern while their loved one is still able to make an informed decision about whether he or she wishes to address these isues in a living will.

CHAPTER 9

The Future

We have described diseases that have beset our species throughout its history. For those who must witness their effects on someone they love, this book promises little immediate relief. We think some of the practical tips we have offered may be helpful, but they only peck at the surface of monstrous tragedies. The hope is for the future, and it lies in biomedical research. Look in that direction and the horizon glows bright indeed.

For perspective, let us briefly review the progress of the brain sciences over the past three decades. Thirty years ago, virtually nothing was known about the brain. Neurotransmission at the junction between nerve and muscle had been studied. The nerve tracks of the spinal cord had been described, and the path taken by messages to and from the lower brain to peripheral structures, such as muscles, had been fairly well worked out. But the brain itself was an unknown black box, or rather a box containing white and gray structures: gray, the bodies of nerve cells; white, the tracks running between gray structures. Every gray and every white feature which could be distinguished had been given a name—medical students memorized every one of the names but knew almost nothing about their features except what to call them. By studying brains damaged by strokes or other injuries, the function of some structures of the brain had been inferred, but in truth our ignorance was abysmal.

We can hardly say that neuroscience research has been marked by a series of brilliant breakthroughs. Rather, progress has been slow and slogging, but it has been steady and it has covered a lot of ground. Today as never before, biology (and perhaps especially the neurosciences) seem poised for a series of advances as dramatic as any in the history of science. In the first edition of this book, we began this chapter with genetics in order to suggest its promise for the future of brain science. In this edition, that entire section has been incorporated into earlier chapters. Its future has come about. Here, then, we can move on to two other technological advances that are enlarging our capacity to study the living brain. We are confident that the next twenty years will see the evolution of a much clearer understanding of the biology of the brain and, we fully believe, the development of effective treatments for progressive dementias.

The first of the technological advances we want to discuss here is positron-emitting tomography.

Positron-Emitting Tomography

Even after a gene, or genes, associated with a disease has been located, and its DNA code discovered, a huge task remains before the information gained can be effectively used. We would still not know the place occupied by the gene's product in the ongoing life processes of the body. What does the protein do? How does it get to where it must do whatever it does? With what other molecules does it work? What environments are associated with changes in the amount of product produced. Such are the questions that await as the physical chemistry of DNA is being unraveled. Answers to them must be found before researchers understand the process well enough to engineer effective interventions into it.

Until recently, holding out hope that we would ever gain that knowledge about the living, functioning human brain required unbridled optimism, unquestioning faith, or both. But it now seems that such optimism and faith were warranted. New techniques have been developed that make it possible to watch the living brain in action. The most dramatic of these techniques is widely known as positron-emitting tomography (PET).

The positron is a positively charged electron with a very short life in nature. As soon as it encounters an electron, which is negatively charged, both types of electrons are destroyed and two photons are produced. The two photons have a peculiar property. As soon as they are produced, they depart from one another at the speed of light in almost exactly opposite directions. Their combined path is therefore a straight line. In research applications, positrons are attached to substances used by brain tissue such as oxygen or glucose. When such substances are administered to a subject, his or her brain will emit photons from areas that are using oxygen or glucose. And the greater the concentration of oxygen or glucose, the greater the number of photons released.

PET technology depends on the foregoing physical properties. The positron–electron collision produces two photons, which instantaneously depart from each other in opposite directions; their path deviates little from a continuous straight line. The subject's head is surrounded by materials that can detect photons, and the detecting materials are so arranged that only simultaneous hits by two photons are recorded. This makes it possible, with essential help from computers, to calculate a line, located with reference to the anatomy of the brain and skull, along which a given positron was destroyed. After a few such lines have been generated, a location at which they cross can be determined, thus pinpointing an area of metabolic activity within the brain.

In current application, the patient's head is surrounded by individual detectors arranged in three to five layers, or arrays. Each layer can produce a separate image of photon emission, so the brain can be seen at different levels, much as computerized axial tomography (CAT scan) permits. Each layer contains over 300 individual detectors. The images produced show the relative amounts of positron-containing substance at specific locations in brain tissue with resolutions now approaching the size of small brain structures.

In the case of glucose or oxygen, the PET scan image reflects the brain's overall metabolic activity. A few preliminary results of studies of progressive dementias have already been reported. In dementia of the Alzheimer type the activity of the outer parts of the brain is greatly reduced. PET has demonstrated that the brain's metabolic activity first decreases in a particular area (the parietal lobe) on one side or the other. The decreasing activity then spreads to other parts of the brain, but the side that was first affected continues to be more severely affected.

In contrast to dementia of the Alzheimer type, Huntington's disease is characterized by normal activity in the outer parts of the brain while certain internal structures (the caudate nuclei) show diminished activity. Such findings are important clues, and they suggest that PET may one day help with diagnosis.

The great promise of PET, however, lies in labeling with positrons, substances involved in specific reactions rather than in overall energy metabolism. This ability will eventually enable investigators to make fine distinctions and elucidate the brain's most subtle reactions. In order to do this, scientists will have to be able to label, with positrons, other substances important to brain function. Choline is a possibility; so are other raw materials used by the brain, such as the amino acid tryptophan. Hormones are likely targets. So are drugs. Using such labeled materials as probes may slowly render the functioning brain accessible to analysis.

Magnetic Resonance Imaging

PET is not the only new technology emerging from the laboratories that promises to help us dissect brain function. Another is magnetic resonance imaging (MRI), which exploits strong magnetic fields to yield detailed three-dimensional replicas of solid objects, including the brain. The image produced depends on the chemical and physical properties of the material being scanned. The process is very sensitive to small changes in these properties; gray matter can actually be distinguished from white matter in images of the living brain.

At present, MRI is being explored mainly though studies of anatomical changes in living brain tissue. It produces extremely clear detailed images that are already proving useful in diagnosis. However, the promise of the technique extends far beyond illumination of brain anatomy. MRI images can be based on several different kinds of physical and chemical information. Therefore, several different images of the same subject can be produced, all containing different information. By choosing suitable chemicals to produce images, investigators hope to come to understand fundamental metabolic processes in living subjects.

A new, relatively simple imaging system, called Single Photon Emission Computed Tomography (SPECT) has been under active development. Early reports suggest that its output is comparable to the quality of PET. If this output proves to be consistent, SPECT offers great advantages over PET. It is much less expensive—so much so that it could be widely installed in research laboratories or, if it proves useful in diagnosis, in hospitals.

The wonder of the new imaging technology to those who have followed the neurosciences is the promise they offer of getting past the skull into the workings of the living brain. Moreover, the techniques seem to be entirely safe to human subjects. There is no reason to expect that MRI will pose biological risks. PET does entail the administration of radioactive material, but the dose is very small and will be reduced further as refinements are made in techniques and equipment.

In any case, positron-emitting compounds have very short half-lives—typically one to two minutes—so the radiation does not persist.

The major drawback is expense. A PET installation can easily run from two to five million dollars and MRI does not cost much less. In addition, teams of highly qualified professionals are required to operate these extremely complex and sophisticated systems. Biomedical research does cost a lot. But those who pay taxes to support research, or who contribute to organizations such as those described in this book, might find it comforting to reflect that the amounts spent on research are a minute proportion of the amounts now being spent on treatments (which are largely ineffective) and on custodial care. Money spent on support of research is a wise investment in the best humanistic sense. For millions of us, it is our single best hope.

That hope for the development of effective treatments of dementia has substantial support in the results of twin studies. Identical twins have identical genes. Therefore, any difference between members of a pair must be attributed to events that occurred after conception. In dementia of the Alzheimer type, as in most diseases, identical twins do not have identical outcomes. When both members of a pair are affected, their ages at onset differ by an average about 10 years, and some identical twins of affected persons never not develop the disease.

We often reflect on a pair of 62-year-old identical twins from a family whose members are at high risk for Alzheimer's disease. One twin, who is now bedridden, has had Alzheimer's disease for 11 years. Her twin has remained perfectly well. There have been no changes in the unaffected twin's serial CAT scans or in her EEGs, and her psychometric test scores have improved, presumably because of practice. Of course, this vast difference in outcome may not be an effect of environment as we usually think of it. The well twin may simply have had better luck, a favorable draw in the unfolding of some random process, such as one involving gene inactivation. But whatever happened (or did not happen) to her is associated with ideal mental well-being, despite the fact that she is known to possess a DNA segment associated with early-onset Alzheimer's disease. Moreover, her good health does not depend on drugs or any other medical imposition on normal life. And if some process now unknown has kept the well twin free of disease for 11 years, there is no reason in principle why we cannot attain 22 such years, or 44, and then we are in effect preventing the disease completely. When we understand nature's rules, such a happy result should be attainable for everyone at risk—and that is nearly all of us.

A

Tests Used in Investigations of Possible Dementias

Medical Laboratory Tests

Medical laboratory tests are likely to be ordered by physicians when they are doing a diagnostic workup of a case of dementia. The following list of tests is intended to be only a general guide. The diagnostic trail may branch off because of the results of a physical examination or other investigations, and additional tests to assess specific systems may be ordered. Some of the tests listed may not be needed in particular cases, because other evidence has made it possible to rule out certain problems.

The following tests are often ordered as screens upon the patient's admission to a hospital or as part of a comprehensive outpatient examination. A brief explanation of the purpose for each is given.

COMPLETE BLOOD COUNT (CBC): Will detect anemia or cancers of the blood system. Will focus suspicion on pernicious anemia or chronic infections and lead to further investigations.

URINALYSIS: May detect diabetes and diseases of the kidney or liver. Infections of the urinary system can be especially troublesome in elderly persons.

ELECTROLYTES: Tested in blood serum. These are salts that are present normally in precisely regulated amounts. Abnormalities in their concentration may cause mental symptoms, though not dementia. Their main importance, however, is as an indicator of major disease of other systems, especially of endocrine glands and kidneys.

ENDOCRINE SCREEN: Mainly for abnormalities of the thyroid gland.

SEROLOGIC TESTS: For syphilis, done on blood, or cerebrospinal fluid, or both; for AIDS, currently done only for high risk populations. May become part of the standard dementia workup.

BLOOD UREA NITROGEN (BUN): Screen for kidney disease.

BILIRUBIN: Elevated in liver disease.

GLUCOSE: Elevated in blood when diabetes is present.

The following tests are often administered in addition to the foregoing screens when dementia is being investigated.

ERYTHROCYTE SEDIMENTATION RATE (ESR OR SED RATE): Is generally positive in chronic infections that may otherwise give little evidence of their presence in elderly persons. Will be positive in inflammations of arteries, which may compromise blood supply to the brain.

VITAMINS (IN BLOOD): Blood levels of folic acid, vitamin B_{12}, and nicotinic acid will be deficient in chronic malnutrition due to neglect, alcoholism, or specific metabolic diseases.

BLOOD AND URINE SCREENS FOR DRUGS: Will detect and identify (in some cases days after their administration) minute concentrations of virtually all drugs that are likely to cause trouble.

CEREBRAL SPINAL FLUID (CSF): Syphilis in the brain may not be detected in the blood. Amounts of protein, and sugar and numbers of cells present (normally, no cells are present in CSF) may lead doctors to suspect tumor, infections, or blood vessel disease in the brain, which may lead to further investigative tests.

ENDOCRINE TESTS (FREE THYROXINE, THYROXINE UPTAKE): If screening tests or physical findings contain the smallest hint of endocrine abnormality, other tests are likely to be done.

Psychological Tests

The Wechsler Adult Intelligence Scale

Generally called simply the WAIS, the Wechsler Adult Intelligence Scale is frequently administered when dementia is a diagnostic consideration. The WAIS consists of eleven subtests, each separately scored. Sample questions from various subtests follow:

1   How many wings does a bird have?

2.   What should you do if you see someone forget his book when he leaves a restaurant?

3.   If two buttons cost 15 cents, what will be the cost of a dozen buttons?

4.   In what way are a lion and a tiger alike?

The most direct test of recent memory in the WAIS is the *Digit Span* subtest, which is made up of two parts, *Digits Forward* and *Digits Backward*. The examiner starts by presenting orally three digits—for example, 5, 8, 2. The subject must repeat the digits back immediately. The number of digits is increased by one after each successful trial up to a maximum of nine. The second part of the test requires the subject to reverse the order in which the examiner presented the digits. Thus, for example, "7, 5, 8, 3, 6" requires a response of "6, 3, 8, 5, 7."

In other subtests, blocks must be correctly placed to form a specified design, or pictures of human forms must be correctly assembled. Typically in progressive dementia, the sections depending on memory (such as digit span), and those requiring a more abstract attitude (such as block design), reveal a more severe defect than tests based mainly on previously learned vocabulary.

The Wechsler Memory Scale

Another test that is often used is the Wechsler Memory Scale, which employs the *Digit Span* subtest of the WAIS and additional tests of memory: remembering details from a story recited by the examiner or remembering pairs of words, some related, (for example, rose–flower), and some unrelated,(for example, obey–inch). In the paired-word test, the examiner presents first a list of ten pairs of words and then only the first word of each pair. The subject is asked to supply the second word of the pair.

A Test We Have Devised and Used

In our clinical work we use the following short test, which we have found adequate for the repeated assessment of patients over several years. It incorporates parts of several tests and some features we added as a result of our experience. However, it is useful as a rough guide only. In no way can it be used to replace the complete psychometric battery, professionally administered.

1. Examiner: "I am going to tell you a short story. Remember all that you can about it. Just after I finish, I will ask you to repeat the story back to me. Then, about fifteen minutes after that, I will ask you to repeat the story again. Here is the story:

"An airliner with 106 people on board was on its way to Tulsa from Cleveland. A careless passenger started a small fire with a cigarette in a lavatory. But a very efficient stewardess put the fire out and the plane landed safely."

Award 1 point for each of the following details mentioned:

1.	airliner	5.	fire—cigarette
2.	106 people aboard	6.	lavatory
3.	from Cleveland	7.	efficient stewardess
4.	to Tulsa	8.	safe landing

Normal recall is five to eight details, but more important is how much information is lost over the fifteen minutes that elapse before the test of delayed recall. Normally, no more than one detail is lost. That is, a subject who scores seven on immediate recall normally gets six, seven, or even eight after fifteen minutes. A victim of moderately advanced progressive dementia may only recall a detail or two after fifteen minutes.

2. Examiner: "Subtract 7 from 100." If the answer is "93," the subject is asked to continue subtracting 7's from each successive answer. Award one point for each correct subtraction until 30 is reached or until 10 answers have been given. Although this task may seem simple, any impairment of intellectual functioning is readily apparent as subjects attempt it.

3. Examiner shows subject wristwatch and asks: "What is this?"
Pointing to band—"What is this?"
Pointing to stem—"What is this?"
Pointing to dial—"What is this?"
Pointing to hand—"What is this?"
Award 2 points for each correct answer.

4. The subject is asked to draw the face of a clock set to 11:10. Even in early dementia, those affected have great difficulty placing the minute hand on 2; rather, they often try to place it on 10. Award 10 points if both hands are correctly placed.

5. The subject is shown a card with five unrelated words on it (card, broom, mutton, snarl, haul) and asked to remember the words. The subject is also shown a card with the names of five fruits named on it (pear, apple, orange, plum, apricot). Dementing persons usually do much worse than normals on the list of fruits, presumably because they do not use the relatedness of the objects as memory aids.

Scoring: Award 1 point for each unrelated word and 2 points for each related word recalled both for immediate recall and for recall after fifteen minutes.

It is possible to score 76 points. There is no "normal" score. The test is used only to follow the progress of an illness. Most persons who score in the range of 15 to 25 are so impaired intellectually that they require full-time supervision, but we have seen gravely impaired persons score up to 35 points.

The Alzheimer's Association in the United States

In 1988 the Alzheimer's Disease and Related Disorders Association, Inc. in the United States shortened its name to "Alzheimer's Association" in order to enhance name recognition, while retaining the full name as its official, registered name.

At the time of publication of this book, the Alzheimer's Association had more than 200 chapters in major and mid-size cities in the United States and in some rural areas. For additional information about chapters and services in specific areas, call the toll free number: 1-800-621-0379 (in Illinois, dial 1-800-572-6037).

ALZHEIMER'S ASSOCIATION
70 East Lake Street, Suite 600
Chicago, Illinois 60601
TEL: 312-853-3060
FAX: 312-853-3660

The Alzheimer's Association also offers books, videotapes, and brochures on Alzheimer's disease and related disorders, and on the many aspects of family support and patient care.

A History of the Association

The Alzheimer's Association has provided much of the impetus behind the sweeping biomedical and societal changes that are steadily transforming the outlook for victims of dementing illness. The story of the association's origin and growth is a remarkable one, and we asked Hilda Pridgeon, a founding spirit, to recount it for this book.

Families of victims of a dementia such as Alzheimer's disease have always faced the grim prospect of the long-term deterioration and eventual loss of their loved one, whether in the early 1900s (when Dr. Alois Alzheimer first identified that specific dementia) or in later years. But it was only in the late 1970s that various groups and individuals insisted that families could join together to help each other, to increase public understanding of the disease, and to advocate increased funding for research.

The founding in 1979 of the national Alzheimer's Disease and Related Disorders Association, Inc., now known as the Alzheimer's Association, and its subsequent rapid expansion and development, testify to the fact that a grassroots movement can succeed. The desperate need of those affected for information and support has fueled the growth of the organization from seven small founding groups to a national organization comprising more than 210 local chapters that provide a variety of services to victims of dementia and their families.

Origins of the Association

In Minneapolis and St. Paul, Minnesota, in the spring of 1979, the families of five dementia victims who had been struggling separately to cope with the problems of caring for deteriorating husbands and fathers decided to band together. At that time, few people knew what the diagnosis of presenile dementia or Alzheimer's disease meant, and no resources were available to help.

Initial public meetings of these families brought an overwhelming response from other families and caregivers in the

Twin Cities area. Family members, through their willingness to share their experiences, launched a public awareness campaign for the fledgling organization. The new organization soon began to hear from family members in other states seeking information on the disease, and it began to learn of similar groups in Columbus, Ohio, in San Francisco, California, and in Seattle, Washington.

As word spread of the existence in Minnesota of an association devoted to Alzheimer's disease, calls and letters from across the nation convinced the volunteers of the need for a larger organization. On September 9, 1979, the Minnesota organization hosted a dinner meeting for interested parties attending a national medical conference on Alzheimer's disease in Minneapolis to discuss the formation of a national organization. Within weeks, the National Institute on Aging scheduled an expanded organizational meeting for October 29, 1979, in Washington, D.C. Representatives from two additional Alzheimer's organizations, the Massachusetts Society Against Senility, in Boston, and the Chronic Organic Brain Syndrome Society (COBS), in Pittsburgh, joined those who had met earlier in Minneapolis. Other attendees included interested individuals and Alzheimer's disease researchers and representatives from the National Institute on Aging. The group agreed to organize a national association within the next year and established its mission as family support, education, research, and public policy. At a later meeting, the Association established a beginning organizational structure, elected officers, and named a Medical and Scientific Advisory Board. Chapters became members of the Association with representation on the national board of directors through a regional delegate system.

The Association's leadership was to be challenged through the next few years by the complex task of bringing together groups with diverse ideas about the order of priority of the new organization's goals. With limited resources available, and given the many needs of the estimated 2.5 million victims, the Association had to set priorities. It chose to support beginning research, advocacy, and services to patients and families.

Growth in the number of chapters began immediately, but during the first year, two of the original groups decided to leave the organization. The Family Survival Project, in San Francisco, California, and ASSIST in Seattle, Washington, withdrew in 1980.

Structure and Financial Growth

The financial growth of the Association has been amazingly rapid. The annual national budget rose from $78,000 in 1980 to $17.5 million in 1990. The effective recruitment of leaders and subsequent planning made this financial growth possible. Public board members were chosen from the business and social communities for their influential positions and were commissioned to raise funds for the organization's operations and research. Most public board members also had a family member stricken with dementia, which inspired and sustained their determination to help. This group of board members, enlarged and changed over the years, has been responsible for raising a high percentage of the national office's operating costs. Additional funding for national operations has come from a percentage assessment of funds raised by local chapters.

The Development of Chapters

Most of the early activities of local chapters and the contacts that made their development possible were handled from the Minneapolis–St. Paul chapter until November 1981, when a national office became well established in Chicago. During succeeding years, the rapid increase in the number of chapters began with the major metropolitan areas of the United States but soon spread to mid-size cities and even rural communities. Wherever a group of 25 families agreed to support and organize services for families, a territory was assigned and organizational assistance was provided from the national level.

By 1990, the network had expanded to include 210 local chapters that offer more than 1600 family support groups, general information and referral to community resources, public awareness and educational programs, and local and state advocacy on behalf of patients and families. Chapters range from well-staffed, metropolitan organizations to smaller, largely volunteer-operated centers. Throughout the chapter network, more than 50,000 dedicated volunteers operate "help lines" for families, lead support groups, and (through chapter boards) actively support new programs. At the national level, the addition of specialized staff and field representatives to assist regional delegates has contributed to the growth of the chapter network.

Patient and Family Services

Early in the development of the organization, the national leadership was concerned about patient care, particularly in nursing homes. It has since expanded those concerns to include other care and family issues, primarily in the area of respite care. In communities where chapters found little or no respite care services, many sought to provide day care and in-home respite for families. Others have worked in cooperation with community groups to initiate and improve respite care and to provide training for respite care workers. (Further information on respite care can be found in the index.)

The National Respite Care Demonstration Program (NRCDP) was established by the Association in 1986 to assist chapters further in developing demonstration respite projects. Recognizing the immensity of the task of providing sufficient respite care to meet patient and family needs, the Association sought to foster further community development of services through grants to chapters. Additional demonstration projects have been funded through a joint venture between the Association, the Robert Wood Johnson Foundation, and the U.S. Administration on Aging.

Autopsy Assistance Network

Another service available to families is assistance in planning for brain autopsy. The Autopsy Assistance Network is a nationwide network of trained volunteers who provide families with information about autopsy and help them obtain a confirmed diagnosis in order to validate death records for purposes of clinical and epidemiological research.

Education

The Alzheimer's Association has provided informational materials for a growing audience of caregivers, medical professionals, and members of the general public. It publishes a national newsletter and has developed a series of brochures on such aspects of the disease as memory failure, diagnosis, care at home, legal issues, concerns of caregivers, and arranging for an autopsy.

The Association has distributed several books on the dementias, including *The 36-Hour Day* by Nancy Mace and Dr. Peter V. Rabins (Baltimore, MD: Johns Hopkins University Press, 1981); *Understanding Alzheimer's Disease,* edited by Miriam K. Aronson (New York: Scribners, 1987); and the first edition of *Dementia: A Practical Guide to Alzheimer's Disease and Related Illnesses* by Dr. Leonard L. Heston and June A. White (New York: W. H. Freeman, 1983). In 1985, the Association, in cooperation with the American Health Care Association, published *Care of Alzheimer's Patients: A Manual for Nursing Home Staff* by Lisa P. Gwyther, ACSW. More recently the organization has developed a series of videotapes on caregiving that are designed to assist families and caregiving professionals.

Public Awareness

When the Alzheimer's Association began, the average citizen had never heard of the disease and would have recognized the symptoms only as something called "senility." The fact that

Alzheimer's disease is recognized as a medical disease today is due in part to the Association's efforts to increase public awareness.

One of the first breakthroughs in nationwide publicity came in 1980, when the "Dear Abby" column referred readers to the Association and gave its address. This occurred soon after the first staff person had been hired in New York City. The overwhelming response of 25,000 letters requesting information gave the new organization some inkling of the need for information. Control Data Corporation helped the organization develop a national mailing list and, for the first few years donated the computer time required for producing labels until the Association became able to buy its own computers.

Individual stories about families dealing with Alzheimer's disease began to appear in national publications. Television documentaries brought the issue into homes nationwide. The movie "Do You Remember Love?" which starred Joanne Woodward and Richard Kiley, though a fictional account, raised public concern about the disease.

In 1982 President Reagan declared a National Alzheimer's Disease week. The next year, through the efforts of volunteers from California to New York, Congress designated November as National Alzheimer's Disease Month, and the Association began an annual publicity campaign to increase awareness.

In 1983, a toll-free national 800 line (1-800-621-0379 or, in Illinois, 1-800-572-6037) was established to handle calls for information ranging from "Where is the nearest chapter?" to "How do we arrange for an autopsy?" By 1989, calls to the 800 line were averaging 37,000 a year.

In 1987, the Association shortened its name to the Alzheimer's Association and chose "Someone to Stand by You" as its slogan. Working on a *pro bono* basis, Leo Burnett USA, a Chicago-based advertising agency, developed an intensive awareness campaign. The campaign highlighted the new slogan and a new Association logo: two persons standing side by side representing the "H" in Alzheimer's. This campaign featured the song "Stand by Me," donated and sung by Ben E. King.

Advocacy and Public Policy

The Association has always given high priority to federal funding of research of Alzheimer's disease. Grassroots advocacy has become very important, not only in increasing funding for research but also in promoting Congressional awareness of the needs of patients and families.

In 1980, several family and professional board members testified at a joint hearing of the Senate Subcommittee on Aging; the Committee on Labor, Health, and Human Services; and the Education Subcommittee of the Appropriations Committee, chaired by Senator Thomas Eagleton. Senator Eagleton called attention to the numbers of patients with dementia and warned of future increases unless the issues of research and care were addressed. Thus began a ten-year effort to promote increased research funding and legislation to help families.

In 1979, federal funding for research into Alzheimer's disease stood at about $9.6 million; by 1983, when the Association launched its first National Program to Conquer Alzheimer's Disease, funding had increased to $22 million. Succeeding years saw gradual increases in research funding to the 1989 level of $130 million.

The first Public Policy Forum in 1989 brought more than 300 people to Washington, D.C., to visit their legislative representatives. This event was repeated in 1990. In 1990, the first Public Policy office was opened with a small staff in Washington, D.C.

During the same period of time in which national advocacy was developing, chapters joined together at state levels to promote legislation to help families in areas of respite care, availability of diagnostic resources, special care units, registries, and autopsy. The appointment of special Alzheimer's disease task forces in at least 23 states has increased the public's awareness of victims' and families' needs and, in many cases, has resulted in legislation. Many volunteers represent the Association on these task forces.

Research

In addition to its efforts to increase federal funding for research, the Association has raised and distributed $18 million for special Alzheimer's Association seed grants, including $10 million through Rita Hayworth Galas and $1.4 million from the chapter network. The purpose of the grants is to encourage interest among researchers in investigating the causes, treatments, and possible cures for Alzheimer's disease and related disorders. Grants are subject to peer review by the Medical and Scientific Advisory Board. The Association's annual report for 1989 indicates that 23 respondents to the original pilot studies, which used $275,000 in seed money from the Association, generated $3.5 million from other sources for additional research.

The Future

The number of people who suffer from Alzheimer's disease and other dementias is now estimated to be close to 4 million. As the population ages, the number of victims will grow, increasing the demand for services and raising many new issues. These issues range from the ravaging costs of long-term care and ethical decisions about prolonging life to possible future diagnostic testing and its value in family and career decisions. The Alzheimer's Association, through its long-range planning and the grassroots efforts of its local chapters, is actively preparing to meet these challenges.

Millions of Alzheimer's disease victims and their families in the United States have benefited from the conviction of those individuals who, a decade ago, believed that their burden could be eased if they worked together. After ten years, many of the following members of the original group still remain active in the Association:

- ○ Miriam Aronson

- ○ Ann Bashkiroff

- ○ Dr. Robert Butler

- Warren Easterly
- Marian Emr
- Martha Fenchak
- Bobbie Glaze
- Dr. Robert Katzman
- Dr. Leopold Liss
- Hilda Pridgeon
- Dr. F. Marrott Sinex
- Jerome H. Stone
- Lonnie Wollin

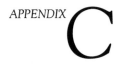

APPENDIX C

ALZHEIMER'S DISEASE
INTERNATIONAL (ADI)

Organized in October 1984, The International Federation of Alzheimer's Disease and Related Disorders Societies, Inc., or ADI, currently includes organizations in the following countries:

ARGENTINA
Association de Lucha contra el Mal de Alzheimer
Hospital Santojanni–Servico Neurologia ALMA
Capital Federal, Buenos Aires
Argentina 1408
TEL: 541-652-0751 and 642-0611

AUSTRALIA
ADARDS (Australia)
P. O. Box 51
North Ryde, N.S.W. 2113
Australia
TEL: 61-2-878-4466
FAX: 61-2-878-4430

BELGIUM
Belgium Alzheimer Liga
Clinic Saint Kamillus
Krijkelberg No.1
3045 Bierbeek, Belgium

TEL: 32-16-46-0496
FAX: 32-16-46-3209

CANADA
Alzheimer's Society of Canada
1320 Yonge Street, Suite 302
Toronto, Ontario M4T 1X2, Canada
TEL: 416-925-3552

ENGLAND
Alzheimer's Disease Society
158–160 Balham High Road
London SW 12 9BN, England
TEL: 01-675-6557 (or 6558,6559,6560)

FINLAND
Alzheimer's Society of Finland
Topeliuksenkatu 17 C
00250 Helsinki, Finland
TEL: 358-0-408-160

FRANCE
France Alzheimer
49 rue Mirabeau
75016 Paris, France
TEL: (1) 45 20 13 26

GERMANY
Alzheimer's Geselschaft
München, E. V.
Mohlstrasse 26
8000 Munich, Germany
TEL: 089-4140-4268

IRELAND
The Alzheimer's Society of Ireland
St. John of God
Stillorgan Co., Dublin, Ireland
TEL: 01-881-282

ITALY
Associazione Italiana Malattia di Alzheimer
Sezione di Milano
Corso di Porta Nuova 32

20121 Milano, Italy
TEL: 0322-800515

MEXICO
Mexican Alzheimer's Association
Irlanda 124
Col. Parque San Andres Coyoacan
Mexico 21, D.F. 04040
TEL: 525-277-3552

NETHERLANDS
Alzheimer Stichting
Postbus 100
3980 CC Bunnik, Netherlands
TEL: 31-3405-96285/96402

NEW ZEALAND
ADARDS (New Zealand)
Box 2808
Christchurch, New Zealand
TEL: (03) 651-590

SCOTLAND
Alzheimer's Disease Society of Scotland
33 Castle Street
Edinburgh, EH2, Scotland
TEL: 44-031-226-3762

SOUTH AFRICA
Alzheimer's and Related Disorders Association
P.O. Box 81183
Parkhurstr, Johannesburg 2120, South Africa
TEL: 011-782-7586

SPAIN
Alzheimer Espana
Alberto Alcocer, 33-5 C
Madrid 28036, Spain

SWEDEN
Alzheimer's Society of Sweden
Sunnanvag 145
S-222 26 Lund, Sweden
TEL: 1646-46-14-7318

SWITZERLAND
Association Alzheimer's Suisse
Route de Florissant 5
CII-1208 Geneva, Switzerland
TEL: 022/47 77 81

VENEZUELA
Fundacion Alzheimer de Venezuela
Santa Capilla a Mijares
Edificio Insbanca Piso 6
Officina 61
Caracas, Venezuela
TEL: 81.92.78-83.89.71

For additional information on ADI, contact:

ADI Deputy Secretary
Alzheimer's Disease International
70 East Lake Street
Chicago, Illinois, U.S.A 60601-5997
TEL: 312-853-3060

The Committee to Combat Huntington's Disease can be reached at the following address:

National CCHD Headquarters
140 West 22 Street
6th Floor
New York, NY 10011
(212) 242-1968

D

Methods of Estimating Risks for Disease from Known Familial Risks

Given the total risk over a lifetime and the distribution of ages at onset, one can estimate the remaining risk at age x from the following equation:

Risk at age x =

$$\frac{\text{risk at birth } (1 - \text{proportion of cases in which illness began by age } x)}{1 - \text{risk at birth} \times \text{proportion of cases in which illness began by age } x}$$

Consider, for example, the Huntington's disease problem described in Chapter 5 and illustrated in Figure 4. We know that 50 percent of the children of a parent with Huntington's disease will themselves develop the disease. We also know that half of those who develop the disease will do so by about age 40. Fitting those numbers into the foregoing equation yields the following risk for the child who is alive and well at age 40, but has a parent with Huntington's disease.

$$\text{Risk remaining at age } 40 = \frac{0.5 \, (1 - 0.5)}{1 - 0.5 \times 0.5} = \frac{0.25}{0.75} = \frac{1}{3} = 0.33$$

The risk at birth (also known as the lifetime risk or the morbid risk) is the risk or probability that a given disease will develop over the lifetime of a person newly born. It is known in some cases from genetic theory; for example, it is 0.5 for Huntington's disease for the child of a parent affected with the disease. For other diseases the risk is *empirically* determined; that is, it is estimated on the basis of accumulated experience with the illness. This is the case with both dementia of the Alzheimer type (DAT) and Pick's disease. The empirical risks for those diseases are given in Tables 7 and 8 that appear in Chapter 5.

For an example of the use of this empirical information, suppose we want to estimate the remaining risk for a person aged 45 whose parent has Pick's disease. Table 8 (see Chapter 5) reveals that the morbid risk for Pick's disease for a first-degree relative of a victim of the disease is 25 percent. From the entries in the table, we may estimate by extrapolation that by age 45, 13 percent of those who will develop the disease have already done so. Then, using the equation given earlier,we estimate the remaining risk for the son or daughter of an affected person who is well at age 45 as:

$$\text{Risk remaining at age } 45 = \frac{0.25\,(1 - 0.13)}{1 - 0.25 \times 0.13} = 0.22$$

To perform the same arithmetic for DAT, use the family types depicted in Figures 5 and 6 and the distribution of ages at onset given in Table 7 in Chapter 5. If a perfect match for family types cannot be found, use the closest one.

One more example: Say we want to know the risk for the daughter of a man who has Huntington's disease and for her son. The daughter will be 28 years old in one month, and she exhibits no sign of Huntington's disease. Her son is 8 years and one month old. Table 6 reveals that the 28-year-old daughter has outlived between 5.4 percent (the proportion affected by age 25) and 13 percent (the proportion affected by age 30) of the total risk of 50 percent. Let us estimate that the daughter has lived through 10 percent of her risk—that estimate is close enough for practical purposes. For the rest of her life, her remaining risk can be estimated as follows:

$$\text{Risk remaining at age 27 years, 11 months} = \frac{0.5\,(1-0.1)}{1-0.5\times 0.1} = 0.47$$

The risk to her son will be one-half of her risk, or 0.235. This is because the son has half of the genes his mother has and, therefore, half as great a chance of having the gene associated with the disease.

Variations of the problems described in this appendix are representative of those that arise in real-life situations. However, many restrictions and caveats may be relevant in any specific case. If there is the slightest doubt about the applicability of the formulas or the estimated risks, consult a genetic counselor. Most major medical centers can refer you to such a person. The stakes are too high to leave room for any doubts about the accuracy of the results you obtain. However, working through specific problems using the foregoing formulas can be most valuable preparation for a visit to a genetic counselor.

Index

ISBN 0-7167-2131-7

EAN

9 780716 721314